GROUP THERAPY

SELF-ESTEEM

Suzanne M. Howard
Certified Mental Health Coach

Battle Press
SATELLITE BEACH, FLORIDA

Group Therapy
Self-Esteem

Books may be ordered through booksellers or by contacting:

Suzanne M. Howard
suzhoward@yahoo.com
www.suzzanehoward.com

Or

Battle Press
steve@battlepress.media
919-218-4039

Because of the dynamic nature of the internet, any web addresses or links contained in this book may have changed since publication and may no longer be valid.

ISBN: 978-1-5136-6576-4 (SC)
ISBN: 978-1-5136-7425-4 (eBook

Library of Congress Control Number: 2021903888

First Edition.

TABLE OF CONTENTS

DEDICATION

To my Dad, Cornelius Karl Dollack,
Who loved me unconditionally.
When he died, that love died with him.
Thus, the journey began...

Self-Esteem & Self-Love
are not given they are grown.

ABOUT THE AUTHOR

Suzanne M Howard is a Certified Mental Health Coach, speaker, Pastor, founder of suzannemhoward.com Coaching, and author of Group Therapy, Self-Esteem, a series of self-help and personal development books.

Suzanne has over a decade of writing curriculums, sermons and speaking throughout the New England region and beyond. She has turned a personal journey into a much broader influence of helping others through their journey. Being a teenage mother in the late 80's, Suzanne has fought, failed and won many battles. She is devoted to her faith and her life long mission to help others overcome their soul issues. She resides in Connecticut with her husband, son and granddaughter.

Suzanne is available for group workshops and one-on-one coaching or mentoring sessions. To learn more please check her out on http://www.suzannemhoward.com or psychologytoday.com.

INTRODUCTION

Most people feel bad about themselves from time to time. The more you like yourself, the more confidence you have. The more you like yourself, the more efficient and effective you are in each area of your life. Self-esteem is the key to peak performance.

Your self-esteem is so important to your emotional health that almost everything you do is aimed at either increasing your feelings of self-esteem and personal value, or protecting it from being diminished by other people or circumstances. Self-esteem, the feeling of liking and respecting yourself, is the foundation principle of success and happiness. It is vital for you to feel fully alive.

You have the right to feel good about yourself. However, it can be very difficult to feel good about yourself when you are under stress or having symptoms that are hard to manage, like dealing with a disability, when you are having a difficult time, or when others are treating you badly. At these times it is easy to be drawn into a downward spiral of lower and lower self-esteem.

For instance, you may begin feeling bad about yourself when someone insults you, when you are under alot of pressure at work, or if you are having a difficult time getting along with someone in your family. Then you begin to give yourself negative self-talk, like "I'm no good." This may make you feel so bad about yourself that you do something to hurt yourself or someone else, such as getting drunk, or yelling at your children. By using the ideas and activities in this book, you can avoid doing things that make you feel even worse, and do those things that will make you feel better about yourself.

Modern day inspirational speakers make it seem like an easy to accomplish task, which it clearly isn't. Building a habit you won't quit on after breaking away from a bad one, and indulging yourself for a period of time, cannot be done by a swish and slash of a wand. More is indeed required.

This book will give you ideas of things you can do to feel better about yourself, which will increase your self-esteem. These ideas have come from people like yourself, people who realize they have low self-esteem and are working to improve it.

As you begin to use the methods in this book and other methods to improve your self-esteem, you may notice feelings of resistance to having positive feelings about yourself. This is normal. Don't let these feelings stop you from feeling good about yourself. They will diminish over time as you feel better and better about yourself. To help relieve these feelings, let your friends know what you are going through. Have a good cry if you can. Do things to relax, such as meditating or taking a nice warm bath.

As you read this book and work on the exercises, keep the following statement in mind:

"I am a very special, unique, and valuable person and I deserve to feel good about myself."

Chapter 1
WHAT IS SELF-ESTEEM?

We all know that self-esteem can be an important part of success. Too little self-esteem can leave people feeling defeated or depressed. It can also lead people to make bad choices, fall into destructive relationships, or fail to live up to their full potential.

Self-esteem is what we think about ourselves. When we think positive we have confidence and self-respect. We are content with ourselves and our abilities, in who we are, and our competence. Self-esteem is relatively stable and enduring, though it can fluctuate. Healthy self-esteem makes us resilient and hopeful about life.

Self-esteem affects not only what we think, but also how we feel and behave. It has significant ramifications for our happiness and enjoyment of life. It considerably affects events in our life, including our relationships, our work and goals, and how we care for ourselves and our children.

Although difficult events such as breakups, illness, or loss of income may in the short term moderate our self-esteem, we soon rebound to think positively about ourselves and our future. Even when we fail, it doesn't diminish our self-esteem. People with healthy self-esteem credit themselves when things go right. When they don't, they consider external causes and also honestly evaluate their mistakes and shortcomings. Then they improve upon them.

What sets Self-Esteem apart from other self-directed traits and states?

---

1. Self-Esteem vs. Self-Concept

Self-esteem is not self-concept, although self-esteem may be a part of self-concept. Self-concept is the perception we have of ourselves, our answer when we ask ourselves the question "Who am I?" It is knowing your own tendencies, thoughts, preferences, habits, hobbies, skills, and areas of weakness.

Put simply, the awareness of who we are is the concept of our self.

---

2. Self-Esteem vs. Self-Image

Another similar term with a different meaning is self-image. Self-image is similar to self-concept in that it is all about how you see yourself. Instead of being based on reality, however, it can be based on false and inaccurate thoughts about ourselves. Our self-image may be close to reality, or far from it, but it is generally not completely in line with objective reality or with the way others perceive us.

---

3. Self-Esteem vs. Self-Worth

Self-esteem is a similar concept to self-worth but with a small (although important) difference. Self-esteem is what we think, feel, and believe about ourselves, while self-worth is the more global recognition that we are valuable human beings worthy of love.

4. Self-Esteem vs. Self-Confidence

Self-esteem is not self-confidence. Self-confidence is about your trust in yourself and your ability to deal with challenges, solve problems, and engage successfully with the world. As you probably noted from this description, self-confidence is based more on external measures of success and value, than the internal measures that contribute to self-esteem. One can have a high levlel of self-confidence, particularly in a certain area or field, but still lack a healthy sense of overall value or self-esteem.

5. Self-Esteem vs. Self-Efficacy

Similar to self-confidence, self-efficacy is also related to self-esteem, but is not a proxy for it. Self-efficacy refers to the belief in one's ability to succeed at certain tasks. You could have high self-efficacy when it comes to playing basketball, but low self-efficacy when it comes to succeeding in math class. Unlike self-esteem, self-efficacy is more specific rather than global, and it is based on external success rather than internal worth.

6. Self-Esteem vs. Self-Compassion

Finally self-esteem is also not self-compassion. Self-compassion centers on how we relate to ourselves, rather than how we judge or perceive ourselves. Being self-compassionate means we are kind and forgiving to ourselves, and we avoid being harsh or overly critical of ourselves. Self-compassion can lead to an healthy sense of self-esteem, but it is not in and of itself self-esteem.

Where Does Self-Esteem Come From?

Once it's clear to you that self-esteem is created by the way you value yourself and your capabilities, it becomes crystal clear that self-esteem comes from you and the thoughts in your brain.

This means that self-esteem does not come from anything that exists outside of you or your mind, like friends and family, or incredible personal achievements.

To appreciate this, let's say that you have extremely supportive friends and family, and every day they tell you that you're the greatest person in the world. You can still have extremely low self-esteem, by still thinking of yourself as a loser, because your self-esteem comes from your thoughts about yourself and not the thoughts or actions of your friends and family.

Similarly, let's say you've achieved amazing things in life, like creating a wonderful family, founding a successful business, running marathons, and so on. You could still have very low self-esteem by thinking very little of those achievements, even though everyone else finds them amazing. It is your thoughts about your capabilities and the achievements that matter, not the achievements themselves.

The lesson, here, is that self-esteem comes from you and the thoughts in your mind, not from anything else. This means that even if you appear to have nothing going for you, you can have extremely high self-esteem, and even if you seem to have everything going for you, you can have very low self-esteem.

It also means that if you want to have higher self-esteem, it's very simple: improve your thinking so that you think more highly of yourself. The fantastic news is that you can change your thoughts very quickly, which means you can swiftly boost your self-esteem.

Chapter 2
PILLARS AND WHY SELF ESTEEM IS IMPORTANT

The Pillars of Self-Esteem:

1. Live Consciously

This first pillar should not come as a surprise. To improve ourselves in any area of life, we first have to become aware of what's going on. There can be no change and no development without first becoming aware of our behaviors, tendencies, and usual responses to certain events.

2. Distinguish Between Fact And Your Emotional Response

Once we practice awareness in our daily life, we will find ourselves in many situations where we allow our emotions to take over and we react very poorly. This has been our "natural" response to these situations for many years, and we have never questioned our behaviors before.

As we start to become aware of our thoughts and behaviors, we can assess our actions. This is important because our natural response is not necessarily the most beneficial.

This is especially true for situations where we get emotionally attached. There are many examples of such situations: meetings where you don't dare to speak up, arguments with your partner which end in huge fights, or conversations with friends. We should use such situations to learn more about our natural tendencies.

---

3. Correct Your Behaviors If Necessary

Awareness is always the first step, but to improve ourselves, we need to correct our behaviors if necessary. There will be cases where it is pretty obvious that our natural response to a situation is not the best solution, like using accusations in a fight with our partner.

---

4. Self-Acceptance

We experience self-esteem, but self-acceptance is something we do.

All of us have likely been in situations where we felt full of self-esteem. This often happens when we are in our comfort zone or doing some activity that puts us into our element. A professional football athlete is likely to feel full of self-esteem on the field, but might not feel very confident in a sales negotiation.

Lack of experience has alot of influence on the level of self-esteem we experience. But while we might not be able to "choose" to be self-confident in certain situations, we can always choose to accept ourselves. We can always choose to value ourselves and to treat ourselves with respect.

Accept that you are what you think, that you desire what you desire, and that you are who you are. Accepting is not judging or liking or disliking. Accepting does not mean we are stuck in this situation. We can still develop ourselves and we are not held back by our thoughts or emotions.

Acceptance is important to create a safe space for ourselves. If we allow ourselves to be who we are, we no longer seek the approval of other people. At this moment, it is okay to be exactly who we are.

This also includes the acceptance of our resistance to the act of accepting facts we don't want to accept. Just remember everything is okay at this moment and can be changed in the future, once we decide to work on it. It is important to remember:

"Acceptance is the Precondition of Change."

---

5. Self-Responsibility

If we want to gain self-esteem, we have to stop seeing ourselves as victims. Being a victim means not being in control and being dependent on others. If our fulfillment lies in the hands of other people, we don't have a chance to gain self-esteem.

Take responsibility for your life, self-fulfillment, and well-being. Taking responsibility is regaining control over our lives. Nobody else will help us in becoming self-fulfilled. We have to stop relying on other people and start relying on ourselves and our power and abilities. You, and only you are responsible for your own well-being, and once you live fully by this principle, nobody else can prevent us from living a fulfilled life. Other people only have as much control over us as we give them.

Concentrate on what is in your circle of influence and neglect what lies outside of it. We are only responsible for the things we can control, and we should also only focus on those aspects. Otherwise, we risk wasting time and energy on things we couldn't control in the first place.

Things inside of your circle of influence include how you respond to situations, the way you take care of yourself, and the way you try to improve your life. This includes exercise, education, meditation, self-love, and much more. Many people believe they need a partner before they can be happy and live a fulfilled life, this is simply not true.

No one is coming to change your life. It is up to you. So instead of waiting for rescue, start taking responsibility for your own life.

---

6. Self-Assertiveness

Assertiveness is a term often associated with negotiations and gaining something you want. Self-assertiveness is a little different, it is more about owning who we are.

---

7. Honor Your Needs And Wants

First, we need to became aware of our behaviors, thoughts, and emotions. Then we can learn to accept who we are, and start to take responsibility for living a fulfilled life.

Now it becomes about honoring our needs and expressing our values. Nowadays, people often call this "Being authentic". It is not only about being honest with ourselves but about what we want and need. It is also about communicating well when interacting with other people. This includes standing behind our ideas and values that might not be so popular with other people. It might also mean to face aversion.

8. Don't Live To Fulfill The Expectations Of Other People

This is easier said than done. In fact, for most people self-sacrifice, and self-surrender are easier than self-assertiveness and standing up for your own needs.

9. Living Purposely

The importance of having goals in life cannot be stressed enough. Having goals gives our life direction. We don't waste our time being unproductive, but rather spend our time becoming an high-achiever. This in itself will lead to an increase in self-esteem.

The goals we choose should be important to ourselves, and independent of other people's opinions or societal standards. Furthermore, it is important to choose specific goals, and not just "I will do my best."

Set a finish date for each goal and make it measurable. Being able to measure your progress toward achieving a goal makes it possible for us to track results and adjust our actions.

Self-discipline is very important. We have to constantly monitor our behaviors and see if those are in line with our goals. Having a goal and working towards it is a great way to prove that we can rely on ourselves.

This is why it is important to stick to our goals once we decide to achieve it, and make an action plan. We don't have to prove anything to anybody else, we only have to prove something to ourselves.

---

10. Personal Integrity

Being the most honest and morally sound version of yourself, gives you personal integriy. We should make this our daily practice.

---

11. Always Make Sure That Your Behaviors Are Congruent To Your Values

When our behavior is consistently in line with our values, we gain more self-esteem, and start to rely on ourselves to take care of our needs and wants. Again, this might lead to situations where we will have to face the aversion of other people, and we might not "fit in." But these are also situations of potential growth.

---

12. Be Honest

Be honest, because anything else is disrespectful to yourself. Lying to gain somebody's approval might feel good at the moment, because we feel accepted by somebody else, but it also includes rejecting ourselves. Everytime we lie, we tell ourselves "we are not good enough." Being honest is huge. We have to be honest, even when it feels uncomfortable. This is especially important when it feels uncomfortable. Remember, only our judgment counts!

Ask yourself this question"What stands in my way of living a life of integrity?" We have to identify the major obstacles and keep on working on them until we live a fully integrated life.

Why Self-Esteem Is Important

Self-esteem is a major factor in people's daily lives, including their routines. Without realizing the impact self-esteem has on us, we have varying levels of it and depend on it daily to perform tasks and activities. Although the meaning of self-esteem is constantly being changed by the way our society views it, it is the basis of one's self-worth and the way we view ourselves.

Self-esteem is important because it greatly influences ones choices and decisions. In other words, self-esteem serves as a motivational function by making it more or less likely that people will take care of themselves and explore their full potential. People with high self-esteem are also people who are motivated to take care of themselves and to persistently strive towards the fulfillment of personal goals and aspirations. People with lower self-esteem don't tend to regard themselves as worthy of happy outcomes, or capable of achieving them, so they tend to let important things slide, and be less persistent and resilient in terms of overcoming adversity. They may have the same kinds of goals as people with higher self-esteem, but they are generally less motivated to pursue them to their conclusion.

Self-esteem can be tough but you can learn to love yourself and cope with your insecurities. Nevertheless, boosting someone else's self-esteem is not an effective way to ensure a healthy and successful individual. I believe that self-esteem is key, and a great foundation for becoming successful in life. I also believe it has to come from the person and not from someone else. Self-esteem isn't given, it's grown. Even though there are ways someone can help, for example, giving you compliments or making you feel loved or happy. These things shouldn't let you feel as if it's boosting your self-esteem. Once those things are gone people lose their self-esteem and feel as if they're worthless.

Before self-esteem was believed to be necessary to one's happiness, the concept seemingly held little or no value to practically anyone. In the past, society didn't have the time or want to focus on something as minuscule as self-esteem -there was much more to worry about such as appearances. Today, however, self-esteem is a key aspect to being truly successful with the life we have all been given, aiding in the advancement of not only our individual lives but what we can do to help further society as a whole. The origin of self-esteem itself has been a huge topic of discussion throughout nations. Dating back to the 1960s, a book by the name of "The Optimistic Child Professor" by Martin Seligman, mentions ways in which self-esteem has a direct correlation to "feeling good". Martin Seligman held the belief that exercises that forcefully try to increase your self-esteem through another person will only result in those people drawing closer to depression.

The Benefits Of Developing Self-Esteem With Meditation

Besides clinical interventions, there are also things people can do on their own to boost their self-esteem. One of these methods is meditation—yes, you can add yet another benefit of meditation to the list! However, not only can we develop self-esteem through meditation, but we can also gain some other important benefits.

When we meditate, we cultivate our ability to let go and keep our thoughts and feelings in perspective. We learn to simply observe instead of actively participating in every little thought or past experience that pops into our heads. In other words, we are "Loosening the grip we have on our sense of self."

While this may sound counterintuitive to developing and maintaining a positive sense of self, it is a great way to approach it. Through meditation, we gain the ability to become aware of our inner experiences without over-identifying with them, and let our thoughts pass by without judgment or strong emotional response.

I enjoy meditating – one of my favorite passages to meditate on is Psalm 23: 1-6:

> [1]*The Lord is my shepherd; I shall not want.* [2]*He makes me lie down in green pastures. He leads me beside still waters.* [3]*He restores my soul. He leads me in paths of righteousness for his name's sake.* [4]*Even though I walk through the valley of the shadow of death, I will fear no evil, for you are with me; your rod and your staff they comfort me.* [5]*You prepare a table before me in the presence of my enemies; you anoint my head with oil; my cup overflows.* [6]*Surely goodness and mercy shall follow me all the days of my life, and I shall dwell in the house of the Lord forever.*

A regular meditation practice can boost your self-esteem by helping you to let go of your preoccupation with yourself, freeing you from being controlled by the thoughts and feelings of your past-experiences. When you can step back and observe a disturbing or self-deprecating thought, it suddenly doesn't have as much power over you as it used to. This de-identification with the negative thoughts you have about yourself results in less negative talk over time, and freedom from your overly critical inner voice.

Chapter 3
FACTORS AFFECTING SELF-ESTEEM

Many factors can influence your self-esteem. Every part of your life can affect it, but the person that has the most control of your self-esteem is you. Start giving yourself good messages about who you are and stop beating yourself up to improve your self-esteem.

Self-esteem plays a significant role in your life. Your self-esteem has a profound impact on the choices you make in your life. It determines what you consider yourself to be capable of and worthy of doing. When you have low self-esteem you are at an higher risk of not fulfilling your real potential in life. Numerous factors can influence your self-esteem. These factors can either build up your self-esteem or pull it down.

---

1. Your Childhood

Your childhood is one of the leading contributing factors to your self-esteem. During your childhood, as your personality and everything else is developing, everyone you encounter has the potential to influence who you become. This influences your self-esteem. For instance, children that grow up in a chaotic home or environment tend to have lower confidence and self-esteem. Children that grow up in unstable homes tend to carry that burden with them throughout their entire lives. All of these childhood experiences can influence to a great extent how they value themselves, even when they are older.

2. Beliefs

Your belief system can either influence your sense of worth positively or negatively. Every family and individual is largely defined by the values and core beliefs that they hold. Some are culturally influenced, while others may be within families, or individually adopted. But they help to define who a person is and will impact how others see them, and how the person sees themself.

Negative beliefs and opinions we hold about ourselves have a big influence on how we see and value ourselves. Some people know that their negative judgment of themselves is too harsh, other people hold onto these beliefs so strongly that they can feel like facts.

3. The Media

Our complete obsession with the media, whether it's social media, television, or print ads, contributes to the widespread self-esteem issues that our society faces. The instant access to social media is especially damaging to young minds with the constant pressure to look and act like public figures, celebrities, and their peers.

4. Friends And Family

The people that you spend time with have a considerable influence on your self-esteem. Your friends can help to build your self-confidence, self-image, and self-respect, or they can bring it down. Unfortunately, there are those in our lives that will purposely try to harm our self-esteem to build themselves up. If your family or friends make you feel unappreciated, not wanted, and undervalued, this can affect how you see yourself and feel about yourself. Your family contributes largely to your self-esteem levels. Family and friends are a major part of the childhood of any person.

Your family can positively or negatively affect your self-esteem. Feelings of inadequacy when it comes to providing for your family can contribute to low self-esteem, while working together as a family and building one another up, can contribute to healthy self-esteem.

---

5. Work Environment

The majority of your time is spent at school or work. The environment tends to influence every aspect of your life, including your self-esteem. If you have a stressful and overly demanding position it can often contribute to low self-esteem. Working in an encouraging and productive environment can have a positive influence on your self-esteem and help you grow stronger.

---

6. Society

The pressure of society to conform to certain standards and ways of living contribute to your low self-esteem. In today's society, there are so many demands for products, fashion styles, and technology. All of these make you feel like you have to live to a certain standard, dress a certain way, have a certain kind of job, and act accordingly. Yielding to this pressure can result in low self-esteem.

7. Relationships

All relationships can influence your self-esteem, but romantic relationships tend to have the biggest effect. Being in a happy and loving relationship can boost your self-esteem. On the other hand, a bad relationship can bring you down in so many ways. A bad breakup or being left by a partner can also weigh heavily on your confidence and self-esteem.

8. Doubting Words From A Loved One

The people in our lives play an important role in developing and nurturing our self-esteem. For example, when our spouse or parents express their joy and pride in our accomplishment, that boosts our self-esteem tremendously. On the other hand, if the same spouse or parents express doubt and concern over our abilities, we begin to doubt ourselves as well.

Thoughts such as 'My mom does not think I am capable of doing this, I can't do it,' or 'My husband does not think I am doing the right thing, so I am wrong,' and so on make us doubt ourselves. Human beings thrive on approval and acceptance from our loved ones, and hence our loved one's opinions can make or break our self-esteem.

Useful Tip:

Be forthcoming to your loved ones and remind them about the huge role they play in your life, and how their support and positivity are important to your well-being. They are your loved ones, and will be happy to provide you with the nourishment that you need.

9. Experience / Situation

People who find themselves in a new situation, or experience something new for the first time may feel unsure of themselves. How they handle the situation can contribute to their self-esteem's growth or decline. People with positive self-esteem generally can handle new situations better. For example, when you walk into a conference room and are not familiar with anyone, people with low self-esteem tend to keep to themselves, or stick with the people they originally find seating with. In contrast, a person with positive self-esteem tends to meet new people and mingle among the crowd with no hesitation.

Chapter 4
REASONS TO BUILD SELF-ESTEEM

"Nobody can go back and start a new beginning, but anyone can start today and make a new ending." Maria Robinson

Nothing is more important than how you feel and think about yourself. Having a high opinion of yourself and knowing who you are, what you do and how much you love yourself are things that people often miss or have too little of in today's society.

But why is building and being able to maintain high self-esteem so important?

Life Becomes Simpler And Lighter

When you like or love yourself more, then things simply become easier. You won't make mountains out of molehills (or out of plain air) nearly as often anymore. You won't drag yourself down or beat yourself up over simple mistakes, or over not reaching a perfect and inhuman standard.

You Will Have More Inner Stability

When you like yourself more, then your opinion of yourself goes up and you'll stop trying so eagerly to get validation and attention from other people

You become less needy, and your inner self becomes much less of a emotional roller coaster based on what people think or say about you today or this week.

Less Self-Sabotage

Most people's worst enemies are themselves. By raising and keeping your self-esteem up you'll feel more deserving of good things in life. And you'll go after them more often, and with more motivation.

When you obtain what you want, then you'll be alot less likely to succumb to self-doubt or self-sabotage in subtle or not so subtle ways.

You Will Be More Attractive In Any Relationship

With better self-esteem, you'll get the benefits listed above. You'll be more stable and able to handle tough times better. You'll be less needy and give more naturally.

Being with you becomes a simpler and lighter experience, with a lot less drama, arguments, or fights based on little or nothing. All of this is attractive in any relationship, no matter if it is with a friend, at work, or with a partner. You'll be happier.

That has been my experience, and is why I write so much about self-esteem. I value my self-esteem so highly and try to keep it steady every day. Because it has made my life so much happier.

But How Do You Practically Improve Your Self-Esteem?

In a nutshell, self-esteem is your opinion of yourself and your abilities. Low self-esteem is unfortunately a self-fulling prophecy. The worse you feel about who you are and what you do, the less motivation you'll have to do what it takes to build your self-esteem.

From there it's easy to spiral down into a cycle of negative and circular thinking, keeping you mired in damaging and erroneous beliefs.

Self-Esteem can be high, low, or somewhere inbetween. While everyone occasionally has doubts about themselves, low self-esteem can leave you feeling insecure and unmotivated. You might be able to identify a few things that are affecting your opinion of yourself (maybe you're being bullied, or you might be feeling lonely), or it could be a mystery.

Either way, if you are wondering how to improve your self-esteem here are steps you can follow on how you do it:

1. Say Stop To Your Inner Critic

A good place to start to increase your self-esteem is by learning how to handle and replace the voice of your inner critic.

We all have an inner critic. It can spur you on to get things done or to do things to gain acceptance from the people in your life. But at the same time, it can drag your self-esteem down. This inner voice whispers or shouts destructive thoughts in your mind.

For example, thoughts like:

- You are lazy and sloppy, now get to work.
- You aren't good at your job at all, and someone will figure that out and throw you out.
- You are worse or uglier than your friend/co-worker/partner.

You don't have to accept this though. There are ways to minimize that critical voice and replace it with more helpful thoughts. You can change how you view yourself.

One way to do so is simply to silence the critic whenever it pipes up in your mind. You can do this by creating a stop-word or stop-phrase. As the critic says something – in your mind – shout: STOP! Or use my favorite: No, no, no, we are not going there! Or come up with a phrase or word that you like that stops the train of thought driven by the inner critic.

Then refocus your thoughts to something more constructive. Like planning what you want to eat for dinner or playing a positive audio book. In the long run, it also helps alot to find better ways to motivate yourself than listening to your inner critic.

---

2. Refocus On Doing What YOU Like To Do

When you like doing something then the motivation to do that thing tends to comes pretty automatically.

When you want something in life then it also becomes easier to push through any inner resistance you feel.

So if you lose your motivation, ask yourself "Am I doing what I want to do?" If not, then refocus and start working on that very important thing instead.

After you have used your stop-word or phrase focus on one of these techniques. Over time it will become a habit and your inner critic will pop up a lot less often.

---

3. Take A 2-Minute Self-Appreciation Break

This is a very simple and fun habit. If you spend just two minutes on it every day for a month then it can make a huge difference.

Here's what you do. Take a deep breath, slow down, and ask yourself this question: "What are 3 things I appreciate about myself?" A few examples that have come up when I use this exercise include:

- I help a lot of people each day.
- I can make people laugh and forget about their troubles.
- I am very thoughtful and caring.

These things don't have to be big:

- You listened fully for a few minutes to someone who needed it today.
- You took a healthy walk or bike ride after work instead of being lazy.
- That you are a caring and kind person in many situations.

These short breaks not only build self-esteem in the long run but can also turn a negative mood to a positive one and reload you with lots of positive energy.

4. Write down 3 Things That You Appreciate About Yourself

This is a variation of the habit above, and combining the two of them can be extra powerful for two boosts in self-esteem a day. You may simply prefer to use this variation at the end of your day when you have some free time for yourself to spare.

Ask yourself the questions from the last section, "What are 3 things I appreciate about myself?" Write down your answers every evening in a journal or on your computer/smartphone.

An extra benefit of writing things down is that after a few weeks you can read through all the answers to help you to stay positive, get a good self-esteem boost, and a change in perspective on days when you may need it the most.

5. Do The Right Thing

When you do what you deep down think is the right thing to do then you raise and strengthen your self-esteem. It might be a small thing like getting up from the couch and going to the gym. Or It could be to show understanding instead of being judgmental in a situation. Or to stop worrying or feeling sorry for yourself, and focus on the opportunities and be grateful for what you have.

It is not always easy to do. Or even to know what the right thing is. But being focused and doing the best you can will make a big difference, both in the results you get, and how you think about yourself.

Useful Tip:

It is easier to stay consistent with doing the right thing if you take several such actions early in the day. Some examples include: giving someone a compliment, eating a healthy breakfast and working out.

---

6. Replace The Perfectionism

Few thought habits can be as destructive in daily life as perfectionism. It can paralyze you from taking action because you become so afraid of not living up to some standard. So you procrastinate and you do not get the results you want. This will make your self-esteem sink. Or you take action, but are never or very rarely satisfied with what you accomplished and how you performed. This lowers your opinion of yourself, your feelings about yourself become more and more negative, and your motivation to take action plummets.

How can you overcome perfectionism? Go for good enough. When you aim for perfection then it usually winds up in a project or a task never being finished. So simply go for good enough instead. Don't use it as an excuse to slack off, but simply realize that there is something called good enough and when you are there then you are finished.

Remember that buying into myths of perfection will hurt you and the people in your life. The simple reminder that life is not like a movie, a song, or book can be a good reality check whenever you are daydreaming of perfection.

7. Be Nice To Yourself

That little voice inside that tells you you're killin' it (or not) is way more powerful than you might think. Make an effort to be kind to yourself. If you do slip up, try to challenge any negative thoughts. A good rule of thumb is to speak to yourself in the same way that you'd speak to your friends. This can be hard at first, but practice makes perfect.

This is because reality can clash with your expectations when they are out of this world, and harm or even lead to the end of relationships, jobs, or projects, and so on.

8. Handle Mistakes And Failures More Positively

If you go outside of your comfort zone or try to accomplish anything truly meaningful, then you will stumble and fall along the way. And that is OK. It is normal. It is what people who accomplished something that truly mattered have done throughout all ages. Even if we don't always hear about it as much as we hear about their successes.

When you stumble try this: Be your own best friend. Instead of beating yourself up, ask yourself, "How would my friend, parent or mentor support me and help me in this situation?" Then do things and talk to yourself like he or she would. This keeps you from falling into a pit of despair and helps you to be more constructive after the first initial pain of a mistake or failure starts to dissipate. Always find the upside.

Another way to be more constructive in this kind of situation is to focus on optimism and opportunities. Ask yourself, "what is one thing I can learn from this" and "what is one opportunity I can find in this situation?"

Following this course of action will help you to change your viewpoint and hopefully not hit the same bump further down the road.

9. Be Kinder Towards Other People

When you are kinder towards others you tend to treat and think of yourself more kindly too. The way you treat other people is how they tend to treat you in the long run. So focus on being kind in your daily life.

- Just be there and listen as you let someone vent.
- Hold the door for the next person.
- Let someone into your lane while driving.
- Encourage a friend or family member when they are uncertain or unmotivated.
- Take a few minutes to help someone out in a practical way.
- Share what has helped you in a difficult situation on social media or a podcast.

10. Try Something New

When you try something new or challenge yourself in a small or big way, and go outside of your comfort zone, then your opinion of yourself goes up.

You may not have done whatever you did in a spectacular or great way, but you at least tried instead of sitting on your hands and doing nothing. That is something to appreciate about yourself. It can help you come alive as you get out of a rut.

So go outside of your comfort zone regularly. Don't expect anything, just tell yourself that you will try something out. Then, later on you can do the same thing a few more times and improve your performance.

As always, if it feels too scary or uncomfortable then don't beat yourself up. Take a smaller step forward instead by gently nudging yourself into motion.

---

11. Do What Makes You Happy

If you spend time doing the things you enjoy you're more likely to think positively. Try to schedule "me" time every day. Whether it's time spent reading, cooking, or just conking out on the couch for a bit, if it makes you happy, make time for it.

---

12. Welcome Failure As Part Of Growth

It's a common response to be hard on yourself when you've failed. But if you can shift your thinking and understand that failure is an opportunity to learn and plays a necessary role in learning and growth, it can help you keep perspective. Remember that failure means you're making an effort.

When you compare your life to other people's lives, and what they have, then you have a destructive habit on your hands. Because you can never win. There is always someone who has more or is better than you at something in the world. There are always people ahead of you.

So replace that habit with something better. Look at how far you have come instead. Compare yourself to yourself. Focus on you and on your results and how you have improved. This will both motivate you and raise your self-esteem.

---

13. Spend More Time With Supportive People And Less Time With Destructive People

Even If you focus on being kinder towards other people and yourself, and on replacing your perfectionism habit, it will still be hard to keep your self-esteem up if the most important influences in your life drag it down on a daily or weekly basis.

So make changes in the input you get. Choose to spend less time with people who are nervous perfectionists, unkind or unsupportive of your dreams or goals. Spend more time with positive uplifting people who have more human and kinder standards, and ways of thinking about things.

Think about what you read, listen to and watch. Spend less time on an internet forum, reading a magazine, or watching a TV-show, if you feel it makes you unsure of yourself. If it makes you feel more negatively towards yourself, then spend the time used on this source by reading self-help or goal-oriented books, blogs and podcasts that help you and that make you feel good about yourself.

14. List Your Accomplishments

Think about all of the things you've accomplished. Make a list of everything you've done and feel proud of everything you've done well. Review your list when you need to remind yourself of your ability to get things done and continue to add to it.

Chapter 5
ELEMENTS OF BUILDING SELF-ESTEEM

To perform at your best and feel terrific about yourself, you should be in a perpetual state of self-esteem building and maintenance. Just as you take responsibility for your level of physical fitness, you need to take complete responsibility for the content and quality of your mind.

I have listed a simple formula that contains all the critical elements of self-esteem building. You can use it regularly to assure maximum performance. The formula is comprised of six basic elements: goals, standards, successful experiences, comparison with others, recognition, and rewards. Let's take them one at a time.

Element One - Goals

How much you like and respect yourself is directly affected by your goals. The very act of setting big, challenging goals for yourself and making written plans of action to achieve them raises your self-esteem, which causes you to feel much better about yourself.

Self-esteem is a condition you experience when you are moving step-by-step toward the accomplishment of something important to you. For this reason, it's really important to have clear goals for each part of your life, and to continually work toward achieving those goals. Each progressive step causes your self-esteem to increase and makes you feel more positive and effective in everything else you do.

Element Two - Standards

The second element in self-esteem building is having clear standards and values to which you are committed. Men and women with high self-esteem are very clear about what they believe in. The higher your values and ideals are, and the more committed you are to living your life consistent with those values and ideals, the more you will like and respect yourself and the higher your self-esteem will be.

Lasting self-esteem comes only when your goals and your values are congruent, that is when they fit with each other like a hand in a glove. Much of the stress that people experience comes from believing one thing and trying to do another. But when your goals and values are in harmony with each other, you will feel a wonderful surge of energy and well-being, and that's when you start to make real progress.

Many people tell me they are unhappy with their job because they can't seem to achieve success, no matter how hard they try. I always ask them if they are doing what they care about and believe in. In many cases, people realize that they are not happy with their job because it is the wrong kind of work for them. Once they change jobs and start doing something they enjoy that is more consistent with their innermost convictions, they begin to make real progress and get a lot of satisfaction out of their work.

Element Three – Successful Experiences

The third element in self-esteem building involves having

successful experiences. Once you have set your goals and standards, you must make them measurable so that you can keep score of your small and large successes along the way.

The very act of setting up a goal and breaking it down into smaller parts, then completing those parts, makes you feel like a winner and causes your self-esteem to increase. Remember that you can't hit a target you can't see. You won't feel like a winner unless you lay out the standards by which you are going to measure your success, and then achieve those standards.

For example, let's say you set a goal to earn a certain amount of income in a given year. If you break this goal down into monthly and weekly goals, and then you achieve the first milestone you will feel great about yourself. Each time you reach another milestone, your self-esteem and ability to perform will increase, and you will feel encouraged and enthusiastic about the next challenge.

Element Four – Comparison With Others

The fourth element of self-esteem building is to compare yourself with others. Leon Festinger of Harvard University concluded that in determining how well we are doing, we should not compare ourselves with abstract standards, but rather, we should compare ourselves with people we know. To feel like a winner, you must know for sure that you are doing as well as or better than someone else. The more you know about how well others in your field are doing, and the more favorably you compare with them, the more you will feel like a winner, and the higher your self-esteem will be.

Successful people continually compare themselves with other successful people. They think about them, read about them and study their performances. Then they work toward surpassing them one step at a time. Eventually, successful people reach the point where they compete only with themselves measured against their past accomplishments. But this comes after they have moved to the top and left many of their competitor's behind.

Element Five - Recognition

The next element for building self-esteem is recognition of your accomplishments by people whom you respect. To feel great about yourself, you need the recognition of people you look up to and admire, such as your boss, your coworkers, your spouse, and people in your social circle.

When you are recognized and praised for any accomplishment by someone whose opinion you hold in high regard, your self-esteem goes up along with your eagerness and enthusiasm to do even better on the job.

Element Six - Rewards

The final element of self-esteem building involves rewards that are consistent with your accomplishments. You may work in a field where you receive financial bonuses, and status symbols like larger offices, bigger cars or even plaques and trophies for superior achievement. All of these symbols can have an incredible impact on raising your self-esteem and causing you to feel terrific about yourself.

Chapter 6
WAYS TO BUILD LASTING SELF-ESTEEM

Many of us recognize the value of improving our feelings of self-worth. When our self-esteem is high, we not only feel better about ourselves, but we are more resilient as well. Brain scan studies demonstrate that when our self-esteem is higher, we are more likely to experience common emotional wounds such as rejection and failure as being less painful, and bounce back from them more quickly. When our self-esteem is high we are also less vulnerable to anxiety, we release less cortisol into our bloodstream when under stress, and it is less likely to linger in our system.

But as wonderful as it is to have a higher self-esteem, it turns out that improving it is no easy task. Despite the endless array of articles, programs, and products promising to enhance our self-esteem, the reality is that many of them do not work, and some are even likely to make us feel worse.

Part of the problem is that our self-esteem is rather unstable to begin with, as it can fluctuate daily, if not hourly. To further complicate matters, our self-esteem is comprised of both our global feelings about ourselves, as well as how we feel about ourselves in the specific domains of our lives, for example as a father, nurse, athlete, etc. The more meaningful a specific domain of self-esteem is, the greater the impact it has on our global self-esteem. Having someone wince when they taste the not-so-delicious dinner he or she prepared will hurt a chef's self-esteem much more than someone for whom cooking is not a significant aspect of their identity.

Suzanne M. Howard

Lastly, having high self-esteem is indeed a good thing, but only in moderation. Very high self-esteem — like that of narcissists — is often quite brittle. Such people might feel great about themselves much of the time, but they also tend to be extremely vulnerable to criticism and negative feedback, and respond to it in ways that stunt their psychological self-growth.

That said, it is certainly possible to improve our self-esteem if we go about it the right way. Here are five ways to nourish your self-esteem when it is low:

---

1. Use Positive Affirmations Correctly

Positive affirmations such as "I am going to be a great success!" are extremely popular, but they have one critical problem — they tend to make people with low self-worth feel worse about themselves. Why? Because when our self-esteem is low such declarations are simply too contrary to our existing beliefs. Ironically, positive affirmations do work for one subset of people — those whose self-esteem is already high. For affirmations to work when your self-esteem is lagging, tweak them to make them more believable. For example, change "I'm going to be a great success!" to "I'm going to persevere until I succeed!"

---

2. Identify Your Competencies And Develop Them

Self-esteem is built up by demonstrating real ability and achievement in areas of our lives that matter to us. If you pride yourself on being a good cook, throw more dinner parties. If you're a good runner, sign up for races and train for them. In short, figure out your core competencies and find opportunities and careers that accentuate them.

48

3. Learn To Accept Compliments

One of the trickiest aspects of improving self-esteem is that when we feel bad about ourselves we tend to be more resistant to compliments, even though that is when we most need them. So, set yourself the goal to tolerate compliments when you receive them, even if they make you uncomfortable (and they will). The best way to avoid the reflexive reaction of batting away compliments is to prepare a simple set of responses and train yourself to use them automatically whenever you get good feedback (e.g., "Thank you" or "How kind of you to say"). In time, the impulse to deny or rebuff compliments will fade — which will also be an nice indication your self-esteem is getting stronger.

4. Eliminate Self-Criticism And Introduce Self-Compassion

Unfortunately, when our self-esteem is low we are likely to damage it even further by being self-critical. Since our goal is to enhance our self-esteem, we need to substitute self-criticism (which is almost always entirely useless even when it feels compelling) with self-compassion. Specifically, whenever your self-critical inner monologue kicks in, ask yourself what you would say to a dear friend if they were in your situation (we tend to be much more compassionate to friends than we are to ourselves) and direct those comments to yourself. Doing so will avoid damaging your self-esteem further with critical thoughts, and help build it up instead.

5. Affirm Your Real Worth

The following exercise has been demonstrated to help revive your self-esteem after it has sustained a blow. Write down a list of your qualities that are meaningful in that specific context. For example, if you get rejected by your date, list qualities that make you a good relationship prospect (for example, being loyal or emotionally available), or if you failed to get a work promotion list the qualities that make you a valuable employee, for example, you have a strong work ethic or are responsible. Then choose one of the items on your list and write a brief essay (one to two paragraphs) about why the quality is valuable and likely to be appreciated by other people in the future. Do the exercise every day for a week or whenever you **need** a self-esteem boost.

Chapter 7
THE FOUR TYPES OF SELF-ESTEEM

As we have said, self-esteem needs to be nurtured, in varying degrees, from the outside. Although the bases are built during childhood, self-esteem is not unalterable in other stages of life.

There are two main types of self-esteem; "High", and "Low". It is important to emphasize that self-esteem is not the same as self-confidence. Self-confidence (also called self-efficacy) is related to the specific goals and objectives that we propose, while self-esteem refers to the global assessment of how we feel about ourselves.

Self-efficacy refers to the confidence in the ability of oneself for a specific task or goal. You could be very good at something and still have low self-esteem. Though you are very good at something, low self-esteem could make you wish you were taller, smarter or have a better physique. On the contrary, self-efficacy could positively affect the self-esteem of the individual if they consider it a priority in their life.

The Four Types of Self-Esteem Include:

---

1. High And Stable Self-Esteem

External circumstances and life events have little influence on self-esteem. People with high and stable self-esteem unfold openly. Since they don't need to defend their image they defend themselves.

Also, the person can defend their point of view without being destabilized.

---

2. High But Unstable Self-Esteem

People with high and unstable self-esteem have high self-esteem but are unable to keep it constant. Competitive contexts can have a destabilizing effect. They respond with a critical attitude to failure, since these are perceived as threats. The individual will show conviction in defending his point of view, but will not accept other points of view and tends to monopolize discussions.

Unstable self-esteem leads to placing self-esteem as a central concern and requires preserving it at any price and appealing to an aggressive attitude (to promote it) or a passive one (to protect it).

---

3. Low And Stable Self-Esteem

In cases where there is low and stable self-esteem, external events (whether favorable or not) do not alter the self-esteem of the subject.

Individuals with this type of self-esteem have a hard time making decisions and have a great fear of being wrong. They do not defend their points of view since the valuation of themselves is always negative, and they believe that they are not up to par.

This type of self-esteem is very common in people with depressive tendencies. Because of their pessimistic mentality they do not usually perceive their achievements based on their own abilities, assuming that they are the result of luck or chance.

4. Low But Unstable Self-Esteem

People with this low and unstable self-esteem are usually sensitive and easily influenced by external events. When they are successful in a certain event their self-esteem rises, but as soon as the euphoria of the moment ends, their level of self-esteem drops again. This type of self-esteem is defined by its lack of solidity and the instability that it presents, which makes them highly sensitive to all types of events however irrelevant they may seem, from a rational point of view.

Certain classes of narcissistic people are characterized by having low self-esteem, and are very dependent on the opinions they perceive from others.

Bonus: Inflated Self-Esteem

Other authors also speak of a type of self-esteem that is detrimental to well-being called inflated self-esteem. But what is inflated self-esteem?

A person with inflated self-esteem is unable to listen to others much less, accept or recognize they made a mistake. Their perception of themselves is so inflated that they think they are better than others. When things get complicated, they do not recognize their mistakes and blame others. This type of attitude generates negative behaviors since they are not capable of self-criticism and correcting their mistakes. In general, these individuals disparage others and adopt hostile behavior toward them.

Chapter 8
LOW SELF ESTEEM

Low self-esteem can be defined as the lack of self-confidence in oneself, or seeing oneself as unworthy, inadequate, incompetent, unacceptable or unlovable. Having negative self-critical thoughts can affect one's behavior and life choices, leaving them trapped in a lonely, vicious circle.

Low self-esteem can also affect one's mental health, leading to stress, depression, and eating disorders. As such, it's important to take quick actions when you realize that you or someone you love is suffering from this debilitating problem.

Having low self-esteem can also be detrimental to your physical health, and negatively affect your personal and professional relationships. There are many reasons why you may have low self-esteem, for example genetics, how and where you grew up, and other life circumstances all play a role.

Low self-esteem generally occurs when a person lacks an appropriate level of self-respect. People with low self-esteem usually feel insecure despite any reassurance they may receive from others. They may find themselves emphasizing their flaws and failures while downgrading their successes and positive attributes. They may harbor negative self-beliefs and speak very negatively about themselves to others. Low self-esteem can increase the risk of mental illness, affect relationships, and damage the overall quality of life.

Most experts believe that low self-esteem develops very early in life, often in childhood or adolescence. One's early relationships with parents, siblings, peers and authority figures are believed to have a massive effect on self-esteem. Those who experience loving supportive relationships early in life are more likely to enjoy healthy self-esteem. Those who experience rejection or abuse whether emotional or physical in early relationships are generally considered less capable of developing a healthy sense of self-worth.

The perceptions of others are considered vital to developing self-esteem. Most children and adolescents look to family, friends, and peers to give them a sense of self-worth. People who develop low self-esteem are often those who feel that they failed in some important way early in life. Many people who develop problems with inadequate self-esteem feel that they have failed to earn the approval of an important person in their lives, such as a parent or partner, and therefore may perceive themselves as inadequate or worthless.

Unhealthy low self-esteem can have several negative ramifications. It is often linked to depression, anxiety disorders, eating disorders, or substance-abuse problems. People who lack an appropriate sense of self-worth may have trouble succeeding at school or work, since they often remain convinced that any efforts they make will lead to failure. Having a low self-opinion of oneself makes it difficult to listen to, or take credit from positive feedback. People with low self-esteem tend to discount any positive feedback out of hand since they are usually quite certain of their negative self-beliefs.

Problems Caused By Low Self-Esteem:

1. You Hate Yourself

While there are times when we all dislike who we are, loathing what you think and the actions you take is a classic sign of low self-esteem. Self-hate is characterized by feelings of anger and frustration about who you are and an inability to forgive yourself for even the smallest of mistakes.

Turn self-hatred around by taking the following actions:

- **Change Your Internal Dialogue.** An internal critic fuels self-hate so the first step is to silence the voice in your head by consciously making yourself repeat a positive response for every negative thought you have. Why be your own worst critic? If you wouldn't say it to your best friend, don't say it to yourself.
- **Forgive Yourself For Your Mistakes.** No one is all good or all bad. Doing something you regret doesn't make you an awful person, just as doing something well doesn't make you a saint.
- **Challenge Your Negative Self-Beliefs.** It's likely that your sense of who you are is outdated and has been passed to you by others, such as your parents, ex-partners, and colleagues. Don't be afraid to rewrite your script – it's your life.

---

2. You Are Obsessed With Being 'Perfect'

Perfectionism is one of the more destructive aspects of low self-esteem. A perfectionist is someone who lives with a constant sense of failure because their achievements, no matter how impressive, don't ever feel quite good enough.

To combat perfectionism:

- **Set Realistic Expectations For Yourself.** Consciously think about how reasonable and manageable your goals are before striving for them, remembering that life in general is imperfect.
- **Recognize The Difference Between Failing And Being a Failure.** There is a huge difference between failing at something you do and being a failure as a person. Don't confuse the two.

- **Stop Sweating The Small Stuff.** Perfectionists' tend to nitpick at insignificant problems. They forget to view the bigger picture and take pride in their accomplishments.

3. You Hate Your Body

A negative body image is often linked to low self-esteem and vice versa. This means it can affect everything from how you behave in relationships to how you project yourself at work. It can even prevent you from looking after your health, because you feel unworthy.

Ways to love your body include:

- **Avoid Comparing Yourself To Others.** Comparison is the thief of joy and only leads to insecurity. Accept that everyone is different and remember where your strengths lie.
- **Look After Your Health.** Following a healthy diet and practicing a daily exercise regime not only makes you feel physically more able but also leads to the release of endorphins, the body's feel-good hormones.
- **Take Care Of Your Appearance.** People with a poor body image often stop making an effort, believing there is 'No point'. Take three positive actions today to improve your looks.

4. You Believe You Bring Nothing To The Table

We all doubt our ability in certain areas of our lives, but a deep-rooted sense of worthlessness comes from believing that somehow we are not as valuable as others. If this sounds familiar, it's important to understand that feeling worthy isn't something given to us by others, but something we have to build ourselves.

To feel more confident about your abilities:

- **Accept We All Have Unique Talents.** We must take pride in our abilities and innate talents to believe we are worthy people.
- **Stop Thinking Others Are Better Than You.** While it's fine to think highly of others, it's irrational to translate this as meaning they are 'better' than you. Admire others' traits, but not at the expense of your own.
- **Be Aware That We Teach Others How To Treat Us**. Practice projecting yourself as someone whose opinions are just as valid as others, and your sense of self-worth will begin to rise.

---

5. You Are Oversensitive

Being too sensitive is one of the more painful aspects of low self-esteem. Whether you're angered by criticism, or feel demolished by any comment that's directed at you, it's important to desensitize yourself.

Strategies for handling criticism include:

- **Listen To What's Being Said.** By listening closely to others you can evaluate whether a comment is true or not, before deciding how you feel about it.
- **Stand Up For Yourself.** If the criticism is unfair, say you disagree.
- **Be Proactive.** If there is some truth in the criticism directed at you, learn from what's being said, rather than beating yourself up about it. Criticism can be constructive, provided you take the comments on board and make changes for the better.
- **Move On**. Replaying over and over what's upset you only anchors the memory to you – which won't help.

6. You Are Fearful And Anxious

Fear and a belief that you are powerless to change anything in your world are irrefutably linked to low self-esteem.

To Combat Anxiety and Fear:

- **Discriminate Between Genuine Fears And Unfounded Ones.** Challenge your anxieties with the facts. For instance, you may feel it's pointless to go for a promotion because you don't think you can get it, however, how true is this statement when you look at the evidence?
- **Build Confidence By Facing Your Fears.** Draw a fear pyramid. Place your biggest fears at the top and your smallest fears at the bottom. The idea is to work your way up the pyramid, taking on each fear and boosting your belief in your abilities as you go.

7. You Often Feel Angry

Anger is a normal emotion but it gets distorted when you have low self-esteem. When you don't think highly of yourself, you start to believe your thoughts and feelings aren't important to others. Repressed hurt and anger can build up so something seemingly small can trigger outbursts of fury.

Healthy ways to express your anger:

- **Learn How To Remain Calm.** Do not let your feelings simmer away until you explode. Instead, express how you are feeling at the time.
- **Remove Yourself.** If the above does not work, step away from the situation and breathe in long slow breaths to reduce your

heart rate and bring your body back to a relaxed state.

- **Don't Overdo It.** People with low self-esteem often over commit, then feel bitter as they struggle to cope. Try to take on only what you want and would like to do.

---

8. You Are A People Pleaser

One of the biggest problems with low self-esteem is feeling you have to please others so that they like, love and respect you. As a result many people-pleasers end up feeling aggrieved and used.

How To Set Personal Boundaries:

- **Learn How To Say No.** Your worth doesn't depend on others' approval, people like and love you for who you are, not what you do for them.
- **Be selfish sometimes.** Or at least think about your needs for a change. People with healthy self-esteem know when it's important to put themselves first.
- **Set limits on others.** Feeling resentful and used stems from accepting things from friends and family that you feel is unacceptable. Start placing limits on what you will and won't do and your resentment will ease.

Sources Of Low Self-Esteem

1. Disapproving Authority Figures

If you grew up hearing that whatever you did wasn't good enough, how are you supposed to grow into an adult with a positive self-image? If you were criticized no matter what you did, or how hard you tried, it becomes difficult to feel confident and comfortable in your own skin. The shame forced on you for perpetually "failing" can feel blindingly painful.

---

2. Uninvolved Or Preoccupied Caregivers

It's difficult to motivate yourself to want more, strive for more, and imagine that you deserve more when your parents or other primary caregivers don't pay attention, and act as if your greatest achievements aren't worth noticing. This scenario often results in feeling forgotten, unacknowledged and unimportant. It can also leave you feeling that you are not accountable to anyone, or you may believe that no one in the here and now is concerned about your whereabouts. This may be carry-over feelings from the past. Feeling unrecognized can result in the belief that you are supposed to apologize for your existence.

---

3. Authority Figures In Conflict

When parents or other caregivers fight or make each other feel bad, children can absorb the negative emotions and distrustful situations that have been modeled for them. It's scary, overwhelming and disorganizing. This experience can also occur when one parent is deeply distraught or acts unpredictably around the child. When you are subjected to excessive conflicts between authority figures, it can feel as if you contributed to the fight and are responsible for your parent's painful circumstance. Intense conflicts are experienced as extremely threatening, and fear driven, leading the child to believe they caused it. This feeling of being "tainted" can be carried into adulthood.

4. Bullying (With Unsupportive Parents)

If you had the support of a relatively safe, responsive, aware family you may have had a better chance of recovering and salvaging your self-esteem after having been taunted and bullied as a child. If you already felt unsafe at home, and the torture continued in the outside world, it can lead to a overwhelming sense of being lost, abandoned, hopeless, and filled with self-loathing pervading your everyday life. It can also feel like anyone who befriends you is doing you a favor because you see yourself as so damaged. Or you may think that anyone involved in your life must be predatory and not to be trusted. Without a supportive home life, the effects of bullying can be magnified and miserably erode the quality of life.

5. Bullying (With Over-Supportive Parents)

Conversely, if your parents were overly and indiscriminately supportive, it can leave you unprepared for the cruel world. Without an initial cause to develop a thick outer layer, it can feel challenging and even shameful to view yourself as unable to withstand the challenges of life outside the home. From this perspective, you may feel ill-prepared and deeply ashamed to admit this dirty ugly secret about you, even to your parents, because you need to protect them from the pain they would endure if they knew. Instead, you hide the painful secret of what's happened to you. Shame can cloud your perspective. Eventually, it can seem as if your parents' opinions conflicts with the world's opinion of you. It can compel you to cling to what is familiar in your life, because it's hard to trust what's real and what isn't. You may question the validity of your parents' positive view of you, and default to the idea that you are not good enough or are victim-like and should be the subject of ridicule.

6. Bullying (With Uninvolved Parents)

If your primary caregivers were otherwise occupied while you were being bullied, and downplayed your experience, or they let you down when you needed their advocacy, you might have struggled with feeling undeserving of notice, unworthy of attention, and are angry at being shortchanged. When the world feels unsafe, shame and pain are brutal. These feelings could also be evoked if parents were in transitional or chaotic states – so that what happened to you wasn't on anyone's radar. If there's chaos at home, it can be hard to ask for attention or to feel like there is room for you to take up space with your struggles. Instead, you may retreat and become more isolated and stuck in shame.

7. Academic Challenges (Without Caregiver Support)

There's nothing like feeling stupid to create low self-esteem. If you felt like you didn't understand what was happening in school as you were getting further and further behind without anyone noticing or stepping in to help you figure out what accommodations you needed, you might have internalized the belief that you are somehow defective. You may feel preoccupied, excessively doubt your smartness, and feel self-conscious about sharing your opinions. The shame of feeling as if you aren't good enough can be difficult to shake, even after you learn ways to accommodate your academic difficulties.

8. Trauma

Physical, sexual, or emotional abuse may be the most striking and overt causes of low self-esteem. Being forced into a physical and emotional position against your will can make it very hard to like the world, trust yourself or trust others, which profoundly impacts self-esteem. It may even feel like it is your fault when it couldn't be less true. Obviously, in these scenarios there is so much going on at one time that you might need to check out, dissociate, or distance yourself. It can make you feel like nothingness. Your brain may have convinced you that you were complicit or even to blame. You may have found ways to cope with the abuse and to manage the chaos in ways that you understand are unhealthy, which ultimately leads you to view yourself as repulsive and seemingly shameful, among a zillion other feelings.

---

9. Belief Systems

When your religious (or other) belief system makes you feel as if you are perpetually sinning it can be similar to the experience of living with a disapproving authority figure. Whether the judgment is emanating from authority figures, or an established belief system in your life, it can evoke shame, guilt, conflict, and self-loathing. Many structured belief systems offer two paths: one that's all good and one that's all bad. When you inevitably fall into the abyss between the two, you end up feeling confused, wrong, disoriented, shameful, fake, and disappointed with yourself over and over again.

---

10. Society And The Media

It's no secret that people in the media are packaged and airbrushed into unrealistic levels of beauty and thinness. It's an epidemic that's only getting worse. Now, males and females alike feel they can't measure up to what's out there. Maybe the seeds of low self-esteem are sown elsewhere, but society and the media make imperfections so immediately accessible, there is no relief from feelings of inadequacy. As media access is available, younger and younger kids are subjected to these unfair comparisons earlier and earlier in life.

Of course, each of these sources of low self-esteem merits an infinite number of posts. It is however most important to understand that experiencing any of these early circumstances doesn't mean you must be bound by them as an adult. They will be woven into your fabric and absorbed into your sense of yourself in different ways over time, but there are many paths to feeling that you are better prepared, less fragmented, and more confident moving forward.

As an adult, when you examine your past history, you can begin to see that in some cases the derision or intense negative messages you encountered weren't necessarily meant for you. Rather, they flowed from the circumstances of the people who delivered them. This perspective can help you to dilute the power of the negative messages about yourself that you received and formed. Furthermore, understanding that you are not alone in your experience can help decrease the extent to which you feel isolated and shameful.

There are some circumstances you have suffered that may be impossible to understand. You can't and aren't expected to understand, empathize, or forgive in these circumstances. What matters most is continuing to find ways to feel OK and as safe as you can in your own life right now. The more you understand the sources of your low self-esteem and can put them into context, the more you can use your self-understanding to begin the process of increasing your self-esteem.

Signs Of Low Self-Esteem

Do you often have a low opinion of yourself? Or consistently think that you're an underachiever and not worthy of compliments or praise? If so, then you could be suffering from low self-esteem. Put simply, self-esteem is how you think about yourself or your overall opinion of yourself. It can also be how you feel about your strengths and weaknesses. Your self-esteem can be high, low, or somewhere in the middle.

There are several signs that either you or someone you know may be struggling with low self-esteem. These signs of low self-esteem include:

1. Sensitive To Criticism

If you have low self-esteem you may be extra sensitive to criticism, whether from others or yourself. You see the criticism only as reinforcing your flaws and confirming that you are incapable of doing anything right.

2. Social Withdrawal

Declining invitations to go to a party or meet up with friends, canceling scheduled plans at the last-minute, and generally not wanting to be around others are signs of low self-esteem. You may not have any desire to hold a conversation or talk about your life because it will only reinforce the depression and anxiety you are already experiencing.

3. Hostility

For someone with low self-esteem lashing out or becoming aggressive towards others is a defense mechanism. If you feel that you are about to be exposed or criticized, attacking whoever might criticize you can be a sign of low self-esteem.

4. Excessive Preoccupation With Personal Problems

Consistently worrying about your issues takes up lots of time for someone with low self-esteem. You may struggle to help or empathize with someone else's problems because you are too preoccupied with your own.

5. Being A Workaholic

At work expectations are set clearly. Even if there's pressure in the workplace, compared to relationships or the social world where so much is unknown and uncontrollable, work is more straightforward.

It is easier to meet expectations and perform well at work. Therefore, some people with low self-esteem shift their focus to work and put all their energies there.

6. Overachieving Or Underachieving

Many of us have already heard that people with low self-esteem tend to be underachievers as they're too afraid to take on new challenges and not confident enough to fully utilize their talents.

However, there's another extreme. Some of them are too anxious about failure and being rejected, so they will try their very best to be outstanding to prove their worth.

Chapter 9
THE CONSEQUENCES OF HAVING LOW SELF-ESTEEM

Since I was a teenager, I was aware of the things that triggered my low self-esteem and the problems it caused. With this awareness, I could take appropriate actions to stop, minimize, or resolve my problem. In other words, I had control over my low self-esteem issue. I might not have had the best solutions then, but at least I knew it was something that affected my life.

Two Situations That Are Worse Than Having Low Self-Esteem:

1. You don't know that you have low self-esteem or you deny it.

2. You are unaware of the problems caused by low self-esteem.

Low self-esteem can lead to a lot of problems, some of which we aren't even aware of. Understanding the effects it brings allows us to focus on resolving the main issue at hand and tackle many sub-problems in our life at the same time.

This is a more effective way of resolving our life problems.

What Are The Negative Effects Of Low Self-Esteem?

Low self-esteem dictates most of our actions. Something we

perceive as positive may be an effect of low self-esteem too. For example, achievement and success aren't bad to have. But if you are constantly striving for them and you realize you can't stop even if you want to, low self-esteem may be the reason for pushing you so hard.

You may think that pursuing success is in your best interest, but you are doing it to avoid feeling unworthy. So in other words, you are controlled by low self-esteem. Your low self-esteem determines what actions you take, not you.

Here are 11 Consequences of Low Self-Esteem:

---

1. It Can Cause You To Spend Too Much Time At Work

Yes, some employers indeed give their employees too much work to do and set unrealistic deadlines. However, sometimes spending too much time at work could be a result of our low self-esteem. Ask yourself:

- Am I the only person who stays late at work?
- Does my whole life revolve around work?
- Are you afraid of making mistakes or letting someone know you make mistakes?

If so, your low self-esteem may be causing you to stay late at work. People with condition-based low self-esteem rely on their work to make them feel good and significant. They are afraid of letting others know they aren't good enough. So they are perfectionists at work, avoiding making mistakes to cover their defects.

Doing a good job is necessary, but is doing it perfectly necessary?

There's nothing wrong with being perfect. Certain jobs such as those in the medical and airline industry require their employees to comply with the procedures perfectly because lives are at stake. But are you being perfect at things that don't add much value to your work? Are you creating more tasks for yourself so that you can avoid other areas of your life such as relationships or health?

Working late is not a problem, but if working late is not required and you are doing it at the expense of other areas of your life, then that's a problem that needs to be addressed.

---

2. It Can Cause You To Do Other People's Work For Them

When you have low self-esteem, you tend to do other people's work for them. There are several reasons why low self-esteem causes people do this:

- Helping others makes you feel needed and worthy.
- You are so used to putting other people's needs over yours that you can't say no.
- You don't have clear boundaries at work.
- You think you are the only one who can do it (this could also be true for high self-esteem people).

Helping others is not the same as doing their work for them. Helping others is great. But if you are helping someone do what they are supposed to do, then you are crossing a boundary. You can point them in the right direction, teach them, and provide them with resources without doing the work for them. What's more, if you resent doing their work, but you can't say no, then it's because you do not value yourself enough to set boundaries at work.

Lastly, thinking that you are the only one who can do a certain task seems harmless. But the truth is most work can be done by others. If you are a manager or an entrepreneur and you find yourself doing the work which you have delegated, it could be you haven't spent enough time teaching others how to do it. Or perhaps you are just holding onto the job because that makes you feel good and competent.

---

3. It Can Make You Procrastinate And feel Unmotivated At Work

Both procrastination and doing other people's work for them would cause you to stay late at work too. What's ironic is when it comes to helping others with their work, we are so willing and quick to say yes. But when it comes to our work, we tend to procrastinate and feel unmotivated.

On a logical level, I get it, that when we do our job well, we are likely to get recognized for our success. However, on a subconscious level, we don't believe we deserve to be worthy and successful, so we sabotage ourselves by procrastinating.

Our mind is full of contradictions.

We want to do well, but are also afraid of the outcome. What if we put in so much time and effort, and it doesn't turn out good? That will reaffirm that we aren't good enough. Or what if we are successful? That will make us feel uncomfortable too because that's not how we perceive ourselves. Plus, being successful would mean more challenges ahead, which means more risks of revealing our unworthiness. Isn't it better to stay as it is?

You may not even notice your mind is full of these contradictions because they act on a subconscious level. But these contradictions are what cause your actions and inaction.

---

4. For Relationships, It Can Prevent You From Connecting With Others On A Deeper Level

When you have low self-esteem, you feel ashamed of who you are. It is difficult to connect with others on a deeper level because you don't want others to know the vulnerable part of you that you are ashamed of. You distance yourself from others because you are afraid of being hurt or exposed.

No one will understand you when you hide your true self from them.

The disadvantage of hiding your authentic self is it makes you feel disconnected from other people. People don't get to know the real you and that's why no one understands you. You can be in a crowded place, a party or with a group of friends and yet still feel very lonely.

This loneliness is just an effect of low self-esteem. Low self-esteem makes you feel defective internally as though you are the only one who is unworthy. But in reality, many others feel the same way about themselves too. And just like you, they aren't sharing their vulnerability with others, so no one knows.

When you compare your "inside" with other people's "outside", you are bound to feel more unworthy, different, and lonely.

5. It Can Cause You To Have Trust Issues With Yourself And Others

Trust is a big thing in relationships, especially intimate relationships. Imagine this: your partner loves you for who you are. But you, on the other hand, don't think too highly of yourself. How does someone who doesn't believe they are worthy of love, trust that another will love them?

Your mind can't comprehend why someone would love a defective person like you. Whenever your partner compliments you or does something for you out of love, you will naturally be doubting if they are genuine or not. You will constantly seek confirmation from your partner or the things they do. What you end up finding though is "evidence" that he or she doesn't love you.

6. It Can Cause Social Anxiety

Low self-esteem causes anxiety too. When you don't feel good about yourself, very often you are worried about how others will view or judge you too. This creates anxiety and stress when you interact with others. You are afraid of saying the wrong things, being boring, or having nothing to say.

7. Low Self-Esteem Creates A Vicious Cycle Of Anxiety

When you don't perform to your expectations socially, you blame yourself for not being good enough, which in turn creates more anxiety the next time you interact with others.

Improving your social skills and building confidence will help ease some of your anxiety. However, if you don't believe you are worthy enough, you will continue to be too self-conscious and over-sensitive. Whenever someone says or does something, you will think they are talking about you when in reality, they aren't. Or even if they are, they might not be saying something negative about you.

---

8. It makes You Confuse Love With Low Self-Esteem

Having low self-esteem, you expect people to treat you badly.

When people are being nice to you, you feel overjoyed and have unrealistically good feelings for them. This can be easily mistaken as love and also scare people away who might be just interested in being friends with you (at first).

---

9. It Makes You Have A Lower Hand In The Relationship

Because you think your partner is too good for you, you bear things that you shouldn't stand for.

Sometimes you even confuse love with self-esteem. Are you giving in really because you love him or her so much, or do you just dare not to speak up and stand up for yourself?

10. It Makes Your Employers Feel That You Are Not Talented

People with low esteem have gifts, but they don't know how to show them or sell themselves.

Example, during a meeting, they might keep quiet, or during a presentation they speak weakly or during daily conversations they consistently say "sorry" and "maybe" too often. As a result, employers and other colleagues perceive people with low esteem as people without many talents.

11. It Can Lead To Depression

Over time, low self-esteem can lead to depression according to a study done by the University of Basel researcher Psychologist Dr. Lars Madsen added that low self-esteem is "A key factor in both the development and maintenance of depression."

Chapter 10
WAYS TO OVERCOME LOW SELF-ESTEEM

If you are suffering from low self-esteem you may be wondering if it's possible to overcome it and regain self-confidence. Well, the good news is that yes it's possible.

In most cases, low self-esteem is usually learned behavior. This implies that those inadequate feelings of self-worth you're experiencing were taught to you by someone else or started because of you focusing on your negatives. So to change this bad learned behavior, you have to start adopting new beliefs and understanding that nobody is perfect. Here are some tips on how to overcome your low self-esteem and start living a happier life.

1. Make Some Improvements

Many things can lead to low self-esteem. Some of them are not in your control, while others are fully within your power to change. For example, being overweight or having a bad body shape are some of the things you can change and improve your self-esteem.

If you are overweight, for instance, you can start taking up an exercise routine and eating better. When you exercise and eat right, there'll be numerous positive changes in your body both in how you feel and how you look. For some people, this can be a great first step in improving their low self-esteem.

If feeling tired all of the time is one of the things that lower your self-esteem, then you can overcome this by turning off the computer and television a few hours earlier and try to get at least 8 hours of good sleep every night. Create a evening routine that makes it easier for you to unwind at night. Getting adequate sleep will help keep your body and mind healthy. You'll also wake up feeling refreshed and full of energy, which will help you accomplish more throughout the day.

2. Accept Some Flaws

I know that this is easier said than done, but it's a must if you want to overcome low self-esteem. There will always be things about yourself that you don't like. Try to understand that this is true for every other person on earth, no matter how flawless they may seem.

One of the tips for overcoming low self-esteem is to learn to concentrate on your strengths, not your limitations.

3. Try Something New

One common characteristic of people suffering from low self-esteem is the feeling that they are incompetent or performers. They think that they're incapable of accomplishing certain things. Sadly, this is many times a self-fulfilling prophecy. To overcome low self-respect, you must understand that you can do more than you think.

You can start by trying something new like taking a photography or pottery class. You can also try to do something daring like parasailing or skydiving. If you've never meditated before, learn to meditate.

With each new adventure or skill you learn, you will add another notch to your confidence level. With time, you will learn that there is nothing you can't do when you believe in yourself.

4. Talk To Your Low Self-Esteem

I know this might sound a little weird, but it can be effective in overcoming low self-esteem. For example, when you're in a meeting, your low self-esteem may tell you "Shut your mouth, you have nothing worth saying in this meeting." If this happens, silently "respond" to your low self-esteem by saying "Yes, I have an idea, and I'm going to speak it out!" And then do it. Even if others don't receive your idea very well, that does not mean that it wasn't worth sharing.

In beating low self-esteem, don't allow your negative feelings to command you. Stand up to them and overcome them by doing what you think is right for you. And before you even know it, you will have increased your confidence, and be on the road to achieving all of your dreams.

5. Try To Relax

One of the things that contribute to low self-esteem is a constant feeling of stress. When you're stressed, your negative thoughts will take charge, making you focus on your weaknesses instead of your strengths. This will even aggravate your stress and lead to more low self-esteem.

Take time to do something you find relaxing. Practice self-care. Try doing things such as taking a bath, gaming, meditation, singing, indoor dancing, etc. This will reduce your stress and make you feel better.

6. Live In The Now

Another way to overcome low self-esteem is to learn to live in the present and not let the hurts of your past or worries about the future affect your actions. You can achieve this by engaging all of your five senses:

1. Stop and listen to the melodious sounds of birds.
2. Feel the breeze of air on your skin.
3. Smell the roses.
4. Enjoy the beautiful color of the sky.
5. Taste the flavor of your favorite ice cream.

All these will draw your consciousness into the present and help you have the right frame of mind when making day-to-day decisions.

7. Be Kind To Yourself

Why would you be kind to others, but be hard on yourself? One of the tricks for overcoming low self-esteem is to treat yourself just the way you'd treat your best pal: be caring, gentle, and forgiving.

Loving-kindness meditation is one way to sit and take time practicing some love and kindness to yourself.

Sometimes, we may be kind to our friends and family but forget to extend that kindness to ourselves! Accept yourself, love yourself, and feel your self-esteem soar.

8. Appreciate Yourself And Know Where You Shine-In

Self-appreciation and self-acceptance are two different things but are connected. You can't appreciate yourself if you don't accept yourself.

Sit down, examine your life, highlight the areas where you do better, and try to work on those areas. Too many times we choose things we know we can't accomplish, and we spend all our time and effort on them. Instead, know your niche and what you're good at, and then focus your hard work, persistence, and dedication, and persistence on that. We all have areas we don't excel at so stop criticizing when you fail at something.

9. Stop Comparing Yourself With Others

I know society has put expectations on you, but you don't have to meet all of them. If you truly want to overcome low self-esteem, you need to start learning to live your life and not trying to please others. Never compare your achievements with those of others. Instead, set your own goals and boundaries and follow your dreams. Remember that we are all different, and each one of us has something unique to deliver. Once you can learn to stop comparing yourself to others, you can be much happier with yourself.

10. Avoid Self-Bashing

As you try to overcome your low self-esteem, remember that we are all human. Everyone, at some point in their life will make a mistake. Some people make way more than others.

One trick to overcoming low self-esteem is to learn not to beat yourself up when you make mistakes. Instead, learn from that mistake. Store it in your memory and use it to prevent you from repeating the same mistake in the future. Always keep in mind that we all learn from trial and error.

11. Surround Yourself With People With A Positive Mind

What we see and hear about ourselves significantly affects our self-esteem. And sometimes, those things may have a permanent effect. Believe it or not, the people you surround yourself with or interacted with in the past have contributed to the person you are today.

If you are trying to feel good about yourself, why surround yourself with people who hate themselves? Why befriend someone who looks down upon himself or herself or has no dreams, goals, or purpose in life?

Spend time with positive people. Start attending conferences with people who want you to be better and who will push you to do the impossible

12. Get To Know Yourself And Become Your Own Best Friend

Despite your differences, you are valuable and deserve to feel good about yourself. Therefore, spend time alone and take time to get to know yourself, which will allow you to discover where you are unique, special, and worthy, which will help you gain a better appreciation of yourself. You can also try making a list of your achievements and strengths to remind yourself of your feats, and then review it whenever you lack self-esteem and need to feel better about yourself.

This is also a great time to pinpoint and confront any negative views that you have about yourself.

13. Acknowledge Where You Need Change

We all have faults; however, if you don't recognize and acknowledge where you need change, it can keep you stuck in a rut of poor self-esteem, which will only get worse the more you try to run from it. Instead, choose to become aware of and acknowledge where you need change and then put forth the effort to improve it. You can even enlist a good friend or relative for support.

You should also become aware when you are too critical of yourself, and then remind yourself that these are not facts, which will help you avoid negative emotions that can lead to negative self-talk.

14. Give Back

Donating, volunteering, and helping others that are less fortunate, not only helps take the focus off your issues, but it also makes you feel good knowing you are helping others. Studies show that doing more things in your life that you can be proud of increases your self-worth, which helps you feel better about yourself.

In the end, people with a positive self-appreciation are open to improvement and more meaningful experiences, meaning they don't rely on external reinforcements, such as status or income, for self-worth, which enables them to experience more happiness and delight in life. Therefore, be mindful of who you allow into your life as well as the circumstances you allow to dictate your self-worth. You should also be mindful to take care of yourself, including exercise and eating right, to help keep both your body and your mind healthy.

Chapter 11
HIGH SELF-ESTEEM

What is High Self-Esteem? How many times in your life have you wondered what kind of person you are? Have you ever thought about how you treat others or how you treat yourself? Chances are good that if you have and you feel good about it, then you probably are somebody who has some of these characteristics of high self-esteem.

High self-esteem can be defined as someone who is completely honest and okay with who they are as a person. They have a very high sense of confidence, and they are very sure of what they do in their lives.

High self-esteem is a positive assessment a person makes of his character. A person considered to have high self-esteem generally views himself as being proficient and worthy in most respects. In general, self-esteem exemplifies how a person regards himself, and there are many benefits of positive self-esteem. Those with high regard for themselves may be more successful in their careers and enjoy a more enriched life.

So if you have high self-esteem, it just means that you think positively about yourself, and you see a lot of positive value in yourself and your capabilities.

To understand this, consider the following list of high self-esteem examples, where you think the following kinds of thoughts about yourself:

- I'm smart
- I have a lot going for me

- I'm interesting
- I'm attractive
- I'm likable
- I'm talented
- I'm a great person
- I'm valuable and important
- I can achieve incredible things with my life
- I'm successful in achieving things I want to achieve

If you have these kinds of thoughts, you're seeing the positive value in yourself, because of the way you're thinking about yourself. Saying that you have high self-esteem is just a shorthand way of saying that you think in these kind's of ways.

What Causes High-Self-Esteem?

It's helpful to appreciate that what causes high self-esteem is the way you think about yourself. Period.

So don't waste your time, like many people do, looking for 'external' fixes for attaining high self-esteem, like accumulating a lot of wealth, having lots of material possessions, having surgery, having people constantly praise and encourage you, and so on.

Here's the thing: you don't need any of these things to think very positively about yourself and your capabilities.

Think about it: you don't need lots of money to appreciate your amazing personality, what a good friend you are, your sense of humor, fun, and adventure, and so on.

Similarly, you don't need surgery to see attractive qualities and beauty in your looks. If you do decide to get surgery, that's fine, but appreciate that you can already see value in your appearance, and learn to be happy with what you see before you even start changing the way you look.

Furthermore, appreciate that even if the entire world hated you, and everyone told you what an awful, worthless person you are, you could still see lots of positive value in yourself and your capabilities, and no one in the world can stop you from doing that.

This means that you are in a very powerful position because you can have very high self-esteem, no matter where you are in life and no matter what others think of you, simply by choosing to think very positively about yourself and your abilities.

Chapter 12
WAYS TO BUILD HIGH SELF-ESTEEM

1. Make Time To Clarify Your Values

Ultimately, high self-esteem comes from living your life in a way that aligns with your values. On the other hand, if you habitually compromise on your values in the way you think and act, you're setting yourself up for low self-esteem, poor self-worth, and low confidence.

For example, have you made a plan to work out at the gym more regularly? Every time you follow through on that goal, you're training your brain to believe that you are trustworthy and reliable, the kind of person who does what they say they will.

But every time you forget or decide to stay on the couch watching Netflix after a long day of work you're teaching your brain that you're not trustworthy and reliable, that you don't care about what you claim to care about. This is a recipe for low self-esteem.

Of course, following through on our best intentions and commitments to ourselves isn't easy. And one of the biggest reasons people struggle to do it is because their values aren't clear and compelling.

Having clear values means you have a well-defined and compelling vision for what matters most to you. The term values include everything from traditional virtues like honesty and integrity down to more mundane but still important commitments like maintaining your physical health through exercise or spending quality time with good friends.

Here's the Catch, though,

When our values are vague and unclear, they don't exert much motivating pull on us. But the more clear, specific, and compelling our values are, the more drawn to them we are, like gravity.

And when our values exert more pull on us, it becomes easier to act in a way that lines up with them and therefore generates high self-esteem.

So, make a plan to spend time regularly clarifying and elaborating on your values.

Here is what I recommend to most people to get started clarifying their values:

---

2. Get Started Clarifying Your Values

I. Set a weekly recurring appointment in your calendar at a time that's convenient and quiet. I like Mondays. Set a timer on your phone for a fixed amount of time, 20 minutes is a good place to start.

II. Take out a notepad, open a Google Doc, or pull out your journal and just start writing about the things in your life that are most important to you. This could be big things like improving your relationship with your spouse or relatively small things like keeping your workspace organized.

III. For each value you identify, try to be as specific and graphic as possible in describing what it is and why it's important. For example, if you're thinking about the value of staying more organized in your workspace, you might describe how calming and peaceful it feels to show up to a clean desk on Monday morning. Or even more specifically, your plan for moving those drawers of loose paper and documents to a organized file cabinet next week.

IV. Stick with your habit. Nothing needs to come out of these values clarification sessions necessarily. But if you commit to doing them regularly, you'll find yourself much more motivated to follow through on your most important commitments and values. And as a result, you'll find yourself getting closer to high self-esteem.

Knowing your values—really knowing them—means a habit of reflecting on them regularly. Once you know your values and begin aligning your thoughts and actions with them, high self-esteem will not be far behind.

---

3. Shift Your Focus From Outcomes To Growth

People with high self-esteem are usually process-oriented.

This means that even though they may have very specific goals and outcomes they would like to achieve, they don't spend much time and energy thinking about them. Instead, they keep their focus squarely on the process of growth—small things they need to do regularly that keep them moving in the right direction.

For example, successful entrepreneurs may have the goal of building a billion-dollar business, but they probably don't waste alot of time and attention imagining what it will be like to hit the billion-dollar mark.

Instead, they focus on hiring talented employees, developing and refining their products, managing their employees well, etc. In other words, they focus on growing their company a little bit more every day, knowing that if the trend continues they will indeed hit their goal.

This focus on process and growth leads to consistently high self-esteem on a personal level because you're regularly reminded of positive movement, even if that movement is modest in size. But if you spend most of your energy thinking about your outcome, all you're going to feel is that you're not there yet, which eventually becomes discouraging and leads to lower self-esteem.

A practical thing you can do to boost your self-esteem is to practice shifting your focus to the small routines and habits that, if performed regularly, will lead to the desired outcome.

Remember, when it comes to goals and outcomes, take a Set It and Forget It approach. Clarify your goals initially, then spend the rest of your time and energy on the routines and actions that will slowly but surely move you there. Not only will you be more likely to reach your goal in the long run, but your self-esteem will grow along the way.

---

4. Eliminate Negative Self-Talk

Self-talk is exactly what it sounds like—it's how we talk to ourselves in our heads. And how we habitually talk to ourselves has a profound effect on how we habitually feel, including our self-esteem.

We all know that self-talk is a thing, but almost no one is fully aware of the extent of their self-talk and how negative it can sometimes be:

- We mutter about how annoying our fellow drivers are at rush hour: "These idiots do not know anything about driving."
- We rationalize that off-handed comment we made to our husband and why it's silly that he's so mad: "He's way too sensitive. He always has been. I was just making an observation."
- We criticize our coworkers for their performance at the sales meeting: "That's got to be the worst sales presentation I've ever seen."

But it is not just negative self-talk about other people and things that are problematic. Even worse is our negative self-talk about ourselves:

- God, I blew it in that conversation. She probably thinks I'm an idiot now.
- Why am I always so lazy?! Everyone else seems to be able to go to the gym regularly. I just can't get myself off the couch in the evenings.
- Don't be such a jerk! I'm so critical of other people. Why can't I be more compassionate with my friends?

When our self-talk is chronically negative and self-critical, it can lead to us feeling discouraged, anxious, guilty, and even depressed. And if we do this to ourselves for long enough and consistently enough, our self-esteem can take a hit.

Even though we may know intellectually that the overly negative things we say to ourselves aren't true (I know I'm not stupid), if we say them to ourselves over and over again (I'm such an idiot), we're going to feel pretty bad anyway.

5. Cultivate A Habit Of Gratitude

This one is a little unusual, but a consistent pattern I've noticed over the years working as a Life Coach is that people who consistently acknowledge and express their gratitude seem to have fairly high self-esteem.

But more than simply expressing their appreciation from time to time, these people seem to be consistent, and even more specifically, they have certain small habits and routines of gratitude so that being grateful is just a part of their lives.

For example, I had a client who was the primary caretaker for her elderly mother who had severe dementia. Now, if you know anything about either dementia or being a caretaker, you won't be surprised by the fact that this is one of the hardest, most stressful jobs anyone can do. When researcher's want to study the effects of chronic stress, primary caretaker's are the best test subjects.

Anyway, despite the stress and burden—both physical and psychological—of taking care of her mom day in and day out, she made it a point to write down one small thing she appreciated about her mom every single day.

She explained that the small routine helped her more than anything else to stay both sane and compassionate in her very trying work. And it's the second part, here, that's important for building high self-esteem.

Her habit of gratitude helped her stay compassionate toward her mother, and the ability to stay compassionate allowed her to maintain high self-esteem.

I think this connection between compassion and self-esteem is hugely underrated. When we are consistently compassionate, both with ourselves and others, we can't help but hold ourselves in high regard. But consistency is the key, which means it's the habit of gratitude that's essential for building higher self-esteem.

6. Manage Your Expectations Effectively

Having your expectations violated is a set-up for frustration, disappointment, and other strong emotional reactions. And unless your emotion management skills are top-notch, being inundated with strong negative emotions regularly makes it easy to fall into self-esteem crushing bad habits like self-judgment, non-assertive communication, and avoidance or isolation.

On the other hand, one of the best and most often ignored ways to reverse the process above and achieve high self-esteem is to manage your expectations better. When we have fewer and more realistic expectations, we can simply avoid a lot of painful emotional experiences in the first place and all the self-esteem crushers that tend to go with it.

7. Spend More Time With The Right People

The type of people we're surrounded by, day-in and day-out, profoundly affects us, including our self-esteem.

It's not hard to see how low self-esteem gets perpetuated if most of the people around you are cruel, sarcastic, condescending, cold, judgmental, and manipulative.

On the other hand, it should be obvious that high self-esteem is far more likely if most of the people in our lives—especially key relationships like spouses, partners, coworkers, best friend, etc.—are supportive, encouraging, loving, kind, compassionate, and honest.

Of course, the details of how exactly other people affect our self-esteem are somewhat complex. And while a deep-dive into that topic would be interesting, it's beyond the scope of this book.

But more importantly, getting lost in these details can be a distraction from a cold hard truth:

Simply making tough decisions to change the type of people you let into your life is key to generating high self-esteem.

For example: that "best friend" you've had since college who still wants to go out drinking every weekend and guilt trips you into it more than you'd like by leveraging your past relationship to get what they want.

This is exactly the type of relationship that is probably damaging your self-esteem more than you realize. Of course, altering the quality of that relationship or removing that person from your life entirely is difficult. So difficult that most people aren't willing to even though they know deep down it's the right decision.

This conflict between what we know we should do and what we end up doing is exactly the kind of thing that maintains low-self esteem. When your actions conflict with your values, your self-esteem is going to suffer.

On the other hand, when you're willing to make the tough choices in the moment to align your behavior with your values, including cutting out bad relationships, high self-esteem may be a lot closer than you imagine.

---

8. Learn To Be Assertive

In its most traditional form, assertiveness means speaking in a way that's both honest and respectful by asking directly for what you want and saying no firmly to what you don't want.

Assertive communication is the healthy alternative to three more common but ultimately destructive styles of communication:

- **Passive Communication:** Holding back on expressing what you want to appease others. Passive communication usually takes the form of "just going with the flow."
- **Aggressive Communication:** Expressing what you want in a way that is dismissive or disrespectful of the rights of others. Often this takes the form of threats or manipulation.
- **Passive-Aggressive Communication:** Trying to get what you want in a way that superficially appears non-aggressive but really is. Sarcasm is a common form of passive-aggressive communication.

When we habitually use any of the three negative communication styles above we erode our self-esteem.

- In **passive communication**, it suffers because we constantly put off our wants and needs.
- In **aggressive communication**, we end up hurting other people and eventually feeling guilty for it.
- In **passive-aggressive communication**, we typically end up alienating people and becoming isolated and lonely.

On the other hand, while it can be difficult in the beginning, assertive communication leads to high self-esteem because we are aligning our speech with our values (what we genuinely want and need) and we're being respectful of the values of others.

As important as assertive communication is, it's only one aspect of a broader concept of assertiveness as an overall way of being in the world. I know that sounds lofty and complex, but it's not.

It all comes down to the relationship between our actions and our values. If the way we habitually act—either in our physical behavior, our speech, or our thoughts—doesn't match up with our values and aspirations, we're going to feel bad. Whether it takes the form of anxiety, depression, addiction, or some other "issue," the core problem is a misalignment of actions and values.

So, in a broad sense, assertiveness means acting in a way that's true to your values, including not just your speech and communication, but also how you think and how you behave.

Chapter 13
CHARACTERISTICS OF
HIGH SELF-ESTEEM

A lot of us fail to succeed in life because we don't think we have what it takes or we are afraid of getting rejected. We miss opportunities and allow doubts and criticisms to take over our decisions because of our low self-esteem. I will explore the characteristics of high self-esteem and provide tips on how to have it.

Self-esteem is like a continuum from low to high. Rather than having low self-esteem or high self-esteem, it's often somewhere in the middle. Your level of self-esteem can also vary in different life situations and with different people. However, if you want to be successful in life, high self-esteem is always better. Knowing the characteristics of high self-esteem is the first step to increasing your level of self-esteem.

Most people settle for mediocrity and let opportunities pass them by because they are afraid of taking risks or making bold actions. Don't allow yourself to become one of those people! Act now and start putting plans in place to boost your self-esteem!

Here are the Characteristics of People with High Self-Esteem:

1. Leaders With A Clear Vision

People with high self-esteem are leaders. They create their path in life. They make their own choices and trust their judgment. If someone doesn't agree with what they want to achieve in life, they don't feel guilty. They refuse to follow and enjoy carving out their path in the world.

If you feel that you're more of a follower than a leader, ask yourself, "What do I want?" Establish a clear vision in your mind of what you want in each area of your life. Once you have that vision, you will notice more resources and more opportunities to help turn that vision into reality.

---

2. Guided By Strong Principles

People with high self-esteem are guided by a set of strong principles and values. Some of these values might be honesty, trust, integrity, openness, transparency, or giving value to others. These principles and values provide a roadmap for their life. They believe and act on those principles and values, and they are ready to defend them.

---

3. Goal Oriented

People with characteristics of high self-esteem set and achieve short-term and long-term goals. Their goals are aligned with their principles and values.

When setting goals, people with high self-esteem aim high but stay realistic. If they set goals that are not achievable and too challenging they will not achieve them. And if they do this repeatedly, it will take a knock on their self-esteem. Make sure that the goals you set are realistic but also aim high.

People with high self-esteem have an inner drive to succeed.

They know what they want or need, and they focus on getting it.

They live life on their terms and create an action plan. They believe that when you set goals and create a plan for your life, you're carving your life in the direction you want. If you don't create a plan, you can easily and unwittingly become part of someone else's plan.

It's crucial to take action and consistently move towards your goals. When you take action, your confidence improves, and your self-esteem increases.

People with high self-esteem are not lazy and don't procrastinate. They work hard and get things done because they don't get bogged down in doubts or complaints. They realize that the more they focus on getting things done, the higher their level of self-esteem.

Low self-esteem people often procrastinate. They waste energy thinking about all the work they have to do rather than just getting it done.

4. Believe In Themselves

People with characteristics of high self-esteem see themselves as valuable, self-worthy and they know that other people will enjoy spending time with them. They believe that they are equal to others, even if their financial and personal success is lower or higher than other people. They focus on their strengths and don't compare themselves to others.

They trust their judgment and don't feel guilty if someone disagrees with them. They don't criticize themselves and avoid internal negative self-talk.

If you would like to increase your level of self-belief, get rid of limiting beliefs, and replace them with positive, empowering beliefs.

Another great tip is to focus on your strengths. What are your strong points? What are you good at? Also, notice what your weaker points are. Set small goals to address them and take action. As the weaker points improve, your level of self-esteem will increase.

---

5. Problem-Solvers

People with characteristics of high self-esteem know that obstacles are a necessary part of the road to success. They deal with obstacles by focusing on them as little as possible, but just enough to resolve them. Their main focus is still on the goal, the vision, and their guiding principles and values.

They enjoy self-solving problems. Whatever the problem, challenge, or obstacle, people with high self-esteem will find a way to figure it out.

People with high self-esteem naturally believe that they can do it. They take calculated risks, adjust to failure if it happens and ask for help if it's necessary. They're also not afraid of rejection. Rejection is a part of life, and they don't take it personally. If you take rejection personally, that can mean that you are avoiding the risks you need to take to get ahead in life and become successful.

---

6. Take Care Of Themselves

People with characteristics of high self-esteem know how to take care of themselves – physically, mentally, emotionally, and spiritually. They are very resilient, emotionally strong, and able to recognize the role of negative emotions. They are not afraid of anger, guilt, or fear. Instead, they look into the reasons behind these emotions and then address them.

They are comfortable looking at themselves in the mirror, and they have a high degree of self-love and self-respect. Their self-talk is positive, empowering, and energizing.

I encourage you to energize yourself with positive and encouraging self-talk. Remember that you are what you think you are and what you say to yourself. When your thoughts and actions are positive, your body will respond with more energy, strength, and drive.

---

7. Great With People

Among other characteristics, people with high self-esteem don't try to please everyone and they avoid gossip.

They can also separate emotion from a message. When someone's angry with them or upset, they can insulate themselves from the emotion and focus on the message that this person is trying to communicate.

They're also sensitive to other people's feelings and their needs. They are fine with accepting and indulging compliments. When they are struggling with something, they are not afraid to ask for help.

They have effective communication and influencing skills. When something's important, they do their best to influence others to see their point of view.

There are 2 types of people in the world, – people that radiate energy and people that drain your energy. They are radiators rather than drainers.

Here is a tip to help you develop higher self-esteem and get better with people. Surround yourself with positive and successful people to gain some of that energy and motivation. When you're around people with high self-esteem, you become more positive and feel better about yourself.

---

8. Transparent

High self-esteem people are open, honest, and transparent. They speak the truth and embrace honesty with no fear of rejection or any intention to harm another person.

If they do something wrong, they are happy to be responsible, take any blame, and own up to their failings. They are accountable for what they say and what they do.

They can also laugh at themselves and see the funny side. Not taking themselves too seriously, they live with an attitude of humility.

---

9. Flexible

People with characteristics of high self-esteem are comfortable with change and know when it is time to try a different approach. They're not set in their ways, and they can adapt to new technology and new ways of doing things.

---

10. Live In The Present

They know that the past is the past and that they can't change it. They have a positive view of the future and the confidence in making that future happen. They don't worry about the future, and they avoid negative "what if" questions. If they notice them, they come up with a strategy and a plan to address and resolve them.

They understand the difference between the past and the present. Their motto would be "My past doesn't equal the future". They won't think their future depends on their past and see the future as something that they can change and influence right now.

---

11. Enjoy Personal Improvement And Always Be Willing To Learn

People with high self-esteem are constantly working on themselves to be the best they can. That's why whenever you see somebody with high self-esteem they either read books, go to seminars, or talk with other people about ways that they can improve their own lives.

---

12. They Have Learned Who They Are And Live like It

They also learned to deal with who they are. They are confident enough in who they are to be what they want to be without worrying about what other people say, or the way they act towards them. They are free spirits.

---

13. They Understand That People Make Their Own Choices

People with this kind of confidence understand that other people can make choices and they let them make those choices because they believe in other people. They understand that other people's choices could be equally as good.

They decide who they are and don't bend to other's perceptions unless they agree.

People with this kind of confidence don't allow other people to make them feel less than they are. They will not be undone emotionally by someone who is trying to hurt them. People can do anything or try to say anything they want but confidence always wins.

---

14. They Recognize How Emotional The World Is For Others

They also understand that everyone deals with anger, sadness and depression in different ways and they are kind and considerate to those people while they deal with them. This leads to people with high self-esteem having more empathy for other people.

Things High Self-Esteem People Don't Do

Having high self-esteem is important if you are aiming for personal or professional success. Interestingly, most people with high levels of self-esteem act in similar ways. That's why it's often easy to pick them out in a crowd. There's something about the way they hold themselves and speak, isn't there?

We all have different hopes, dreams, experiences, and paths, but confidence has its universal language. This list will present some of the things you won't find yourself doing if you have high self-esteem:

1. Compare Yourself To Others

People with low self-esteem are constantly comparing their situation to others. On the other hand, people with higher self-esteem show empathy and compassion while also protecting their sanity. They know how much they can handle and when they can offer a helping hand.

In the age of social media, however, social comparisons are nearly ubiquitous. One study found that "participants who used Facebook most often had poorer trait self-esteem, and this was mediated by greater exposure to upward social comparisons on social media." You will feel worse about yourself if you are constantly getting glimpses into lives that you consider to be better than yours.

Try to limit your time on social media. Also, when you do start scrolling, keep in mind that each profile is carefully crafted to create the appearance of a perfect life. Check yourself when you find yourself wishing for greener grass.

2. Be Mean-Spirited

People with low self-esteem bully others. They take pleasure in putting other people down. People with positive self-esteem see no need to make others feel bad, choosing instead to encourage and celebrate successes.

If you find that you feel the need to put others down, analyze where that's coming from. If they've had success in life, help them feel good about that achievement. They may do the same for you one day.

3. Let Imperfection Ruin Your Day

Perfectionism isn't necessarily a bad thing, but obsessing over making everything perfect is a sign that you have low self-esteem and can lead to never-ending negative thoughts. This can turn into an inability to solve problems creatively, which will only make self-esteem issues worse.

Those with high self-esteem disconnect from the results and do their best without expecting perfection.

People with that kind of confidence understand that messing up is a part of life, and that each time they aim and miss success, they'll at least learn something along the way.

If you miss the mark, or if your plan doesn't work out exactly as you would have liked, take a deep breath and see if you can pivot to do better next time.

4. Dwell On Failure

It's common to hear people dwelling on all the ways things can go wrong. They are positive that their every failure signals an impossible task or an innate inability to do something. People with healthy self-esteem discover why they failed and try again.

People with higher levels of confidence also tend to adopt a growth mindset. This type of thinking supports the idea that most of your abilities can be improved and altered, as opposed to being fixed.

For example, instead of saying, "I'm just not good at math; that's why I did bad on the test," someone with a growth mindset would say, "Math is difficult for me, so I'll have to put in some more practice to improve next time."

---

5. Devalue Your Self-Esteem

People with high self-esteem value their perception of themselves. They understand that they come first and don't feel guilty about taking care of themselves. They believe charity starts within, and if they don't believe that, they'll never have a healthy self-image.

Self-care is often top of the priority list for people with self-esteem

---

6. Try To Please Others

They can't please all the people all the time, so confident people first focus on doing what will make them feel fulfilled and happy. While they will politely listen to others' thoughts and advice, they know that their goals and dreams have to be completed on their terms.

---

7. Close Yourself Off

Confident people can be vulnerable. It's those with poor self-esteem that hide all the best parts of themselves behind an emotional wall. Instead of keeping the real you a secret, be open and honest in all your dealings.

As Brené Brown, author of *Daring Greatly,* points out, "Vulnerability is about showing up and being seen." When you embrace each facet of who you are and allow others to see them as well, it will create deeper, more meaningful connections in your life. When that happens, you'll realize that perfection doesn't lead to people liking you more.

8. Follow And Avoids Leading

People with low self-esteem don't believe they can lead, so they end up following others, sometimes into unhealthy situations. Rather than seeking a sense of belonging, people with high self-esteem walk their paths and create social circles that build them up.

9. Fish For Compliments

If you're constantly seeking compliments, you're not confident. People with high self-esteem always do their best (and go out of their way to do good deeds) because it's what they want to do, not because they're seeking recognition. If you need to hear compliments, say them to yourself in the mirror. You can even try some positive affirmations if you need a confidence boost.

10. Be Lazy

People work harder when they have high self-esteem because they're not bogged down by doubts and complaints. Those with low self-esteem end up procrastinating and wasting their energy thinking about all the work they have to do rather than rolling up their sleeves and just getting it done.

This may also bounce off perfectionism. Perfectionists often feel intimidated by certain projects if they fear that they won't be able to complete them perfectly. Tap into your confidence and simply do your best without worrying about a perfect outcome.

11. Shy Away From Risks

When you trust yourself, you'll be willing to participate more in life. People with low self-esteem are always on the sidelines, waiting for the perfect moment to jump in. Instead of letting life pass you by, have confidence in your success and take the risks necessary to succeed.

12. Gossip

People with low self-esteem are always in other peoples' business – they're more interested in what everyone else is doing than themselves. People with high self-esteem are more interested in their own lives and stay out of others' affairs.

Instead of participating in idle gossip, talk about some positive news you heard recently, or that fascinating book you just finished. There's plenty to talk about beyond what this or that person did wrong in their life.

Chapter 14
SELF-ESTEEM AND SELF-RESPONSIBILITY

Good self-esteem implies that we have some control over what happens in our lives. This means that we each take responsibility for our decisions, behavior, and achieving our goals.

The bottom line is: No one is going to make our life better or to save us! The more we do for ourselves and look out for ourselves, the higher our self-esteem will be. When we practice self-responsibility, it is an active approach to work and life as opposed to a passive one. If we fail to practice self-responsibility, we allow ourselves to be at the mercy of other people or situations.

Three roles are often played out in the work situation that highlights a lack of self-responsibility: the rescuer, the victim, and the oppressor. None of these individuals take any responsibility for themselves.

The rescuer is the person who either keeps quiet about their true feelings or tries to please everybody else, even if it happens at the expense of their well-being. The rescuer will agree with their senior for fear of being unpopular or disliked. The rescuer feels responsible for keeping other people happy and making life easier for others.

The victim is the person who feels helpless to affect change in situations. This person identifies strongly with the martyr role and automatically looks to themselves to find fault. The victim will feel that no matter what they do, life just does not work out for them. Victims come across as very unsure of themselves and apologetic.

The oppressor is the person who blames everyone around them. They are very good at diverting any attention away from themselves and will be quick to point fingers at other people. They will also use fear tactics to gain cooperation. Oppressors come in different guises: those who are overt bullies and who coerce, manipulate, or humiliate others. Then some are much more subtle in the way they try to manipulate others or butter them up to gain their support.

In consulting with executives and business owners, I have seen how the more experienced and wiser businessmen have learned lessons in their careers. They have learned which battles are worth taking on and which may tarnish their reputation. They have learned how not to be hooked into situations or any of the three roles described. They work hard on either not taking situations personally or working through their feelings of frustration or anger. They have learned to temper their responses.

Younger executives may still find themselves reacting from an emotional state. One of my clients was a director of a Human Resources company who reported into a larger group. Initially, he was almost subservient in his interaction with his seniors. He was always motivating the performance of his company or his behavior.

As we worked on his self-esteem and he felt more confident, he began to see himself as an equal to his seniors. They soon noticed this and started consulting him on decisions affecting the larger group. He moved from being a victim to recognizing his self-worth and stepping into his inner power.

None of the three roles described are helpful at work or in life. It is crucial therefore to know that each of us is responsible for the following:

- The achievement of our desires.
- Our choices and actions: "I am the key change agent in my life".
- The level of consciousness we bring to our work: to do our work well or not, to blame others or take responsibility for ourselves.
- The level of consciousness we bring to our relationships: "Am I fully present in interactions? Do I think of the implications of what I say? Do I notice how others respond to what I say?"
- Our behavior with other people: "How do I speak? How do I listen?"
- Our happiness: "No one else is responsible for making me happy."
- Accepting or choosing values by which we live: "Do I live my values or those of others?"

It is very clear from research I have done with successful executives and business owners that each of them feels very strongly about taking responsibility for themselves and learning from situations.

No one is coming to rescue us and make life easier for us. The onus is on each of us to look with awareness at our life. We need to empower ourselves to make decisions that will serve us and the greater community better in the future.

How to Take Responsibility For Your Life

1. Stop Blaming Other People

The most important step to taking responsibility for your life is to stop blaming others.

Why? Because if you're not taking responsibility for your life, it's almost certain that you're blaming other people or situations for your misfortunes. Whether it's negative relationships, a bad childhood, socio-economic disadvantages, or other hardships that inevitably come with life, it's always something other than yourself that's at fault.

Now don't get me wrong: Life is unfair. Some people have it worse than others. And in some cases, you are the victim.

But even if that's true, what does blaming get you?

The victim card? An illusory advantage of preaching victimhood? Justification for life's unsatisfactory conditions?

In reality, blaming only results in bitterness, resentment, and powerlessness.

The people who you target with blame probably don't care about how you feel, or they have no idea anyway.

The bottom line is this:

Those feelings and thoughts may be justified, but it won't help you become successful or happy.

Letting go of blame doesn't justify other people's unfair actions. It doesn't ignore life's hardships.

But the truth is this:

Your life is not about them. It's about you.

You need to stop blaming so you can reclaim your freedom and power that is yours.

No one can take away your ability to take action and make a

better life for yourself.

It's easy and convenient to blame others, but it does nothing to improve your life in the long run.

All it does is cost you the authority of being in charge of your own life.

---

2. Stop Making Excuses

Making excuses for your choices in life, or excuses about what you feel you have achieved – and what you have not – fuels cognitive bias.

When you make excuses, you don't allow yourself to learn from your mistakes.

After all, no failure or mishap is your fault. It's always something else.

When there's no personal accountability, there's no way to grow. You'll be stuck in the same place complaining and dwelling on negativity without ever moving forward.

When you take responsibility for your life and stop making excuses, you silence the negativity.

You realize that what happens outside yourself doesn't matter.

There's only one thing that matters, and that's your actions.

3. Ask Yourself How Other People Impact You

If you feel like the victim in your own life, you need to stop and think about how you let other people impact your outlook on life.

For example, if someone makes a snide remark about you, logic would dictate that it's a reflection of their self-worth.

But in many cases, we think illogically about these things and feel like we are being attacked.

Your perceptions of others reveal so much about your personality.

A huge suite of negative personality traits is associated with viewing others negatively.

So if you take these results to heart, there is no point in taking things personally.

What people say about you clearly says more about themselves than anything to do with you.

4. Love Yourself

If you're struggling to take responsibility for yourself and your actions, then I'm willing to bet that you don't value yourself, either.

Why?

Because people who have self-esteem problems generally don't take responsibility for their lives. Instead, other people are blamed, and a victim mentality is created. Self-esteem won't be boosted until you wise up and take responsibility.

Responsibility empowers you to take action to improve yourself and help others. And self-esteem goes both ways. If you're relying on external validation like praise from other people to fuel your self-esteem, then you're giving away power to others.

Instead, start building stability within. Value yourself and who you are. When you love yourself, there's no other option but to take responsibility. After all, it's your reality, and the only way to make the most of it is to take responsibility for your actions.

---

5. What Does Your Day Look Like?

A crucial way to take responsibility for your life is with your daily habits.

Are you improving your life? Are you growing?

If you don't look after yourself and your daily you, then it's likely that you're not.

Are you taking care of your body, your mind, and your needs?

Here are all the ways that you could be taking responsibility for your mind and body:

- Sleeping properly
- Eating healthy
- Giving yourself time and space to understand your spirituality
- Exercising regularly
- Thanking yourself and those around you
- Playing when you need it
- Avoiding vices and toxic influences
- Reflecting and meditating

Taking responsibility and loving yourself is more than just a state of mind – it's about actions and habits that you do every single day.

You have to take responsibility for yourself, from the beginning of your day to the end. Accepting negative emotions as part of life is tough for most people to accept. After all, no one wants to experience negative emotions. But if you want to start taking responsibility for yourself you need to take responsibility for your emotions as well.

And the truth is this:

Nobody can be positive all the time. We all have a dark side. If you ignore the darker part of life, then it will come back to bite you even harder later on.

Taking responsibility means accepting your emotions. It's about being honest with who you are.

Listen to your being. It is continuously giving you hints; it is a still, small voice, it does not shout at you. Be the person you are. Never try to be another, and you will become mature. Maturity is accepting the responsibility of being oneself, whatsoever the cost. Risking all to be oneself, that's what maturity is all about.

---

6. Stop Chasing Happiness With Outside Attachments

This is something that isn't easy to realize.

After all, many of us may think that happiness means obtaining a shiny new iPhone or getting a higher promotion at work for more money. It's what society tells us every day! Advertising is everywhere.

But we need to realize that happiness only exists inside ourselves.

Outside attachments give us temporary joy – but when the feeling of excitement and joy is over, we go back to the cycle of wanting that high again. An extreme example highlighting the problems with this is a drug addict. They're happy when they're taking drugs, but miserable and angry when they're not. It's a cycle that no one wants to be lost in.

True happiness can only come from within.

It's time to take power back and realize that we create happiness and inner peace inside ourselves.

---

7. Do What You Say You Will Do

There couldn't be a better phrase for taking responsibility for your life than to do what you'll say you'll do.

Part of getting your act together and taking responsibility for your life means being trustworthy and living your life with integrity.

I mean, how do you feel when someone says they'll do something and they fail to do it? In my eyes, they lose instant credibility.

Don't do the same and lose credibility with yourself.

The bottom line is this: You can't take responsibility if you won't even do what you say you'll do.

So, the question is: How can you make sure to follow up with actions on what you say.

Follow these four principles:

- Never agree to or promise anything unless you are 100% sure you can do it. Treat "yes" as a contract.
- Have a schedule: Every time you say "yes" to someone, or even yourself, put it in a calendar.
- Don't make excuses: Sometimes things happen that are beyond our control. If you're forced to break a commitment, don't make excuses. Own it, and try to make things right in the future.
- Be honest: The truth isn't always easy to say, but if you're not rude about it, it will help everyone out in the long run. Being impeccable with your word means you're honest with yourself and with others. You'll become that guy or girl that people can rely on.

---

8. Stop Complaining

Nobody enjoys hanging around a complainer. By complaining, you cannot accept the present moment and take action. You are wasting precious energy complaining about a situation when you could be taking action.

If you can't take action, what's the point in complaining?

Taking responsibility is all about taking action for your own life. Complaining is the antithesis of that.

---

9. Focus On Taking Action

This is probably the most critical part of taking responsibility for your life. We all have goals and ambitions, but without action, they won't be achieved. And what good is someone who talks about doing things but never does it?

Without taking action, it's impossible to take responsibility.

Even if it's small steps, as long as you're doing the work and moving forward, your life will improve. Remember, taking action starts with your habits. Taking little steps every day results in a big step over an extended period.

10. Hang Out With People Who Don't Bring You Down

A huge part of who you become is who you spend most of your time with.

Here's a great quote from Tim Ferriss:

"But you are the average of the five people you associate with most, so do not underestimate the effects of your pessimistic, unambitious, or disorganized friends. If someone isn't making you stronger, they're making you weaker."

It's your responsibility to choose people that will add to your life. People that encourage you to grow. If you continually hang around toxic people who are always complaining and blaming, you'll eventually do the same. Choose to spend time with people who are mature, responsible, and want to live a productive life.

Not only is hanging out with the right people crucial for your mindset, but it may be a massive predictor for your happiness as well.

Chapter 15
TACTICS TO CHANGE HOW YOU SEE YOURSELF

Your sense of self-worth will impact every arena of your life. Your job, your relationships, and even your physical and mental health are a reflection of your self-esteem. But what exactly helps shape your view of yourself and your abilities? The truth is that your level of self-esteem may have grown or shrunk based on how people have treated you in the past and the evaluations you've made about your life and your choices.

The good news is that you have a fair amount of control when it comes to increasing your level of self-worth. There are simple, concrete changes you can make that challenge your mind and your body. One such change is to take steps to reduce negative thinking and build up positive, encouraging thoughts about the person you are and can be.

Low self-esteem can negatively affect virtually every facet of your life, including your relationships, your job, and your health. But you can boost your self-esteem by taking cues from types of mental health counseling and coaching.

Consider these steps for boosting your self-esteem based upon Cognitive Behavioral Therapy:

1. Replace Negative With Positive Thinking

- **Identify triggers –** To increase the level of positive thinking in your day-to-day life, you first have to recognize what people, places, and things promote negative thinking. Maybe it's the balance in your bank account, or perhaps it's a coworker who's always complaining. You can't change certain situations, but you can change how you react to them and understand them. That starts with paying attention to what makes you feel sad or anxious.

- **Take notes** – There's an ongoing dialogue, or "self-talk", always happening in your brain as you go about your day. This self-talk takes in the world around you and makes evaluations about yourself and others. So take the time to start noticing any interesting trends in this dialogue. Is this thinking based on facts? Or is it usually leaning towards the irrational, always assuming the worst in a situation?

- **Challenge your thinking** – If you see yourself jumping to conclusions or always downplaying the positive about yourself, then you have to step up and add some positive thinking to your self-talk. Learning to focus on the positive and to encourage yourself is a lot like strengthening a muscle. You have to exercise your brain a little every day to develop a capacity for positive thinking, to forgive yourself when you make mistakes, and to learn to give yourself credit when you accomplish a goal.

---

2. Take An Inventory

If you're unsure where you rank when it comes to self-esteem, taking an inventory of your personal qualities can help. If you find yourself listing more weaknesses than strengths, this might be a sign that you tend to be too hard on yourself. Consider what talents, abilities, and passions you have not listed or maybe even discovered yet. Never assume you know everything about yourself and what you're capable of. People with high self-esteem leave room for self-discovery every day.

---

3. Acknowledge Successes

Often people with low self-esteem will dismiss their successes as luck or chance. Or they might focus on not being perfect rather than highlighting how far they have come. People with high self-esteem take the time to celebrate their accomplishments. They say, "Thank you" when people compliment them, rather than dismissing their praise. This doesn't mean that people with high self-esteem are arrogant or narcissistic; they just have faith in their abilities and acknowledge successes when they do happen.

---

4. Stop Comparing Yourself

Other people can't be the standard when it comes to your self-esteem. This is because you'll always find someone who appears better than you or more capable than you in any arena of life. Social media certainly doesn't help, as researchers have found that people who check social media very frequently are more likely to suffer from low self-esteem. Remind yourself that people usually only share the best parts of their life online. Your own life should be the yardstick rather than others' lives because what is your best may not be someone else's, and vice versa. Remind yourself that any time you make an improvement or prevent yourself from repeating a mistake, you are making progress.

---

5. Practice Self-Care

The more you demonstrate that you value your health, the more you develop a capacity for loving other parts of yourself.

Listen to your body and avoid foods that make you feel irritable or tired. Eating healthy and exercising also can increase positive thinking and help you feel more encouraged about your future. If you spend time with people who care about you, you may find that suddenly it's easier for you to care for yourself.

Remember that learning positive thinking and developing healthy lifestyle strategies aren't going to be overnight miracles. Being kind to yourself and increasing your sense of self-worth takes time, practice and patience. But the more you challenge your thoughts and perspectives, the greater joy you can find in yourself and your abilities. You'll feel proud of how far you've come, and you'll look forward to the future.

---

6. Identify Troubling Conditions Or Situations

Think about the conditions or situations that seem to deflate your self-esteem. Common triggers might include:

- A work or school presentation
- A crisis at work or home
- A challenge with a spouse, loved one, co-worker, or other close contacts
- A change in roles or life circumstances, such as a job loss or a child leaving home

---

7. Become Aware Of Thoughts And Beliefs

Once you've identified troubling situations, pay attention to your thoughts about them. This includes what you tell yourself (self-talk) and your interpretation of what the situation means. Your thoughts and beliefs might be positive, negative, or neutral. They might be rational, based on reason or facts, or irrational, based on false ideas.

Ask yourself if these beliefs are true. Would you say them to a friend? If you wouldn't say them to someone else, don't say them to yourself.

---

8. Challenge Negative Or Inaccurate Thinking

Your initial thoughts might not be the only way to view a situation, so test the accuracy of your thoughts. Ask yourself whether your view is consistent with facts and logic or whether other explanations for the situation might be plausible.

Be aware that it can be hard to recognize inaccuracies in thinking. Long-held thoughts and beliefs can feel normal and factual, even though many are just opinions or perceptions.

Also, pay attention to thought patterns that erode self-esteem:

- **All-or-nothing thinking**. You see things as either all good or all bad. For example, "If I don't succeed in this task, I'm a total failure."
- **Mental filtering**. You see only negatives and dwell on them, distorting your view of a person or situation. For example, "I made a mistake on that report and now everyone will realize I'm not up to this job."
- **Converting positives into negatives**. You reject your achievements and other positive experiences by insisting that they don't count. For example, "I only did well on that test because it was so easy."
- **Jumping to negative conclusions**. You reach a negative conclusion when little or no evidence supports it. For example, "My friend hasn't replied to my email, so I must have done

something to make him or her angry."

- **Mistaking feelings for facts**. You confuse feelings or beliefs with facts. For example, "I feel like a failure, so I must be a failure."
- **Negative self-talk**. You undervalue yourself, put yourself down, or use self-deprecating humor. For example, "I don't deserve anything better."

---

9. Adjust Your Thoughts And Beliefs

Now replace negative or inaccurate thoughts with accurate, constructive thoughts.

Try these strategies:

- **Use hopeful statements**. Treat yourself with kindness and encouragement. Instead of thinking your presentation won't go well, try telling yourself things such as, "Even though it's tough, I can handle this situation."
- **Forgive yourself**. Everyone makes mistakes — and mistakes aren't permanent reflections on you as a person. They're isolated moments in time. Tell yourself, "I made a mistake, but that doesn't make me a bad person."
- **Avoid 'should' and 'must' statements**. If you find that your thoughts are full of these words, you might be putting unreasonable demands on yourself — or others. Removing these words from your thoughts can lead to more realistic expectations.
- **Focus on the positive.** Think about the parts of your life that work well. Consider the skills you've used to cope with challenging situations.
- **Consider what you've learned**. If it was a negative experience, what might you do differently the next time to create a more positive outcome?

- **Relabel upsetting thoughts**. You don't need to react negatively to negative thoughts. Instead, think of negative thoughts as signals to try new, healthy patterns. Ask yourself, "What can I think and do to make this less stressful?"
- **Encourage yourself**. Give yourself credit for making positive changes. For example, "My presentation might not have been perfect but my colleagues asked questions and remained engaged which means that I accomplished my goal."

10. Step Back From Your Thoughts

Repeat your negative thoughts many times or write them down in an unusual way, such as with your non-dominant hand. Imagine seeing your negative thoughts written on different objects. You might even sing a song about them in your mind.

These exercises can help you take a step back from thoughts and beliefs that are often automatic and observe them. Instead of trying to change your thoughts, distance yourself from your thoughts. Realize that they are nothing more or less than words.

11. Accept Your Thoughts

Instead of fighting, resisting, or being overwhelmed by negative thoughts or feelings, accept them. You don't have to like them, just allow yourself to feel them.

Negative thoughts don't need to be controlled, changed, or acted upon. Aim to lessen the power of your negative thoughts and their influence on your behavior.

These steps might seem awkward at first, but they'll get

easier with practice. As you begin to recognize the thoughts and beliefs that are contributing to your low self-esteem, you can counter them or change the way you think about them. This will help you accept your value as a person. As your self-esteem increases, your confidence and sense of well-being are likely to soar.

Chapter 16
MYTHS ABOUT SELF-ESTEEM

1. Feeling Bad Can Be Cured By Thinking Positively

One thing that we hear a lot when we are feeling bad is that we should 'think positively'. People never seem to tire of coming out with this particular piece of advice. And yet it's no help to anyone to hear it – the truth of the matter is that if I am depressed and you advise me to try to think positively I will feel worse, not better. Why this should be so is not too hard to understand. If I am feeling down then I am going to be having a negative outlook on life – whoever heard of someone feeling down and yet being optimistic at the same time? This is utter nonsense. Yet people are more-or-less guaranteed to come along and tell me (with nothing but the best intentions, of course) that what I should do is to try to think positive thoughts instead of negative thoughts. But if I could think in an upbeat, positive way then I would not be depressed, and so I would not need you to come along and advise me to think positively.

On the other hand, if I am depressed – and for the sake of the argument we will say that I am – then you coming along and breezily tell me that the way to not be depressed is to try to change my negative thinking into positive thinking this advice is not merely 'unhelpful,' it is downright punishing.

No one wants to be depressed, and if it were as simple as just forcing oneself to think positive thoughts instead of negative ones then obviously no one would ever be depressed. Of course it's good to think positively and not be always seeing the worst side to everything, but if I force myself to think positively then it isn't real. It's only real if it is happening naturally and if it is happening by itself.

We can give many examples to show that this is so. To give just one: if you say you like me without me making you say it, then this is happening naturally and it is worth something, but if you are only saying it because I am making you say it, then it is worthless, it doesn't mean a thing. Everybody knows that. It's the same when I try to force myself to do anything that ought to be spontaneous. This is true for laughter, love, creativity, interest, compassion, and it is also true for happiness. Happiness is a spontaneous thing, a gift from above – we cannot give it to ourselves, and the idea that we can is wrong. Nobody wills themselves to be happy – it just doesn't happen that way. Happiness does not come about as a result of intention and calculated action.

2. Things Will Get Better If I Put On A Happy Face

Another thing we often hear is that if you smile, and put a brave face on things, even when you don't feel like it, then eventually you will feel as good as you are pretending to. Experience shows, however, that this is simply not true.

The opposite is true because the more you deny your true feelings and hide behind a smiling mask, the more unbearably horrible and hollow you will feel inside. In our superficial, image-based society the myth is that if you look good on the outside (by buying expensive designer outfits, having your hair done, having perfectly white teeth, working out in the gym, having plastic surgery done) this will somehow percolate through to the inside and make everything right there.

So, if everything is bright and breezy and full of light on the outside, everything will be grand on the inside. Of course, as soon as we see this written down in black-and-white on a page it doesn't sound quite so convincing. It would be more accurate to say that it starts to sound pretty dumb.

From an intuitive point of view, we are likely to suspect that 'fixing the outside' (which is easy and costs us relatively little) is only a poor substitute for tackling the deeper issues, which is a different kettle of fish entirely. Fixing the outside so that I will be happy on the inside is putting the cart before the horse.

---

3. Low Self-Esteem Can Be Cured By Accepting Yourself

It is often said that the key to overcoming low self-esteem is to 'accept oneself'. If you suffer from what is generally called 'low self-esteem' the chances are that you will hear this quite a lot. It is of course very obviously true that if you accept yourself then you won't have low self-esteem, but telling someone who has low self-esteem to accept themselves is ridiculously unhelpful – it is the same as telling someone who is depressed to try to think positively instead of negatively.

The reason I don't accept myself is that I don't like myself, because I think I'm a crappy person. If I was able to accept myself then that would mean that I was okay about myself, and if I was okay about myself then that would mean that I didn't have low self-esteem, and if this was the case then I wouldn't need to try to 'accept myself' in the first place! There is another way of looking at why the advice to 'accept yourself' is not helpful. Any deliberate act of will, any purposeful, goal-orientated action, always involves accepting the outcome that you want and rejecting the outcome that you don't want. This is inherent in the very nature of goal-orientated action.

What this means is that any purposeful action equally involves acceptance and rejection – these are the two sides of the coin, one can't exist without the other.

---

4. It Is Important To Love Yourself

Another thing that we hear a lot is that we need to learn to 'love ourselves'. People say that being able to love yourself is an essential part of good mental health. The trouble is that trying to love me is the same as trying to accept myself which means that when I try to implement this 'first step' I straightaway tie myself up in knots. It is an impossible instruction. And if this weren't enough of a problem, there is also the problem that practically none of us understands what that word 'love' really means.

Of course, we all function based on attachments and that is perfectly normal. But this does not mean that we should kid ourselves that attachments are anything other than attachments. That doesn't mean that we should validate them or justify them and say to ourselves that they are 'the way to go'.

We are all fundamentally selfish and this is perfectly normal – but that does not mean we should go around claiming that selfishness is the same thing as caring about others. Because we don't understand what love is when people say that it is important to love yourself. This is bound to be interpreted as 'be attached to yourself'.

5. Good Self-Esteem Is The Result Of Achievement

The idea that the way to overcome low self-esteem is by achieving is a classic 'mental health myth'. Like all the other myths that we have looked at, it seems to make perfectly good sense when we hear it, but when we think about it more deeply we can see serious problems with it.

When I look around I can see that people have different degrees of confidence in themselves, and it is easy to think that the amount of self-confidence someone has depends on how much they have achieved in life. Achievement seems to be the magic word. This idea fits in with the 'it's good to be a winner' ethos that we are brought up on from childhood. The hidden message in our culture – reinforced by a constant barrage from the mass media – is that it's good to win and bad to lose, and so the answer to everything is simply to be a winner.

Winning is by its very nature competitive, which means putting yourself above everyone else and being happy when you get the good stuff rather than them. This is of course purely and ignorantly self-centered – and yet somehow this crudely self-centered attitude is supposed to make us feel happy!

This message might be unashamedly crass and shallow but that doesn't alter the fact that, deep down, we all tend to believe it. How could we not believe it, given the fact that we hear this message, in innumerable disguised variants, hundreds of times every day? Believing that 'winning is what counts in the end' is the same as believing that 'money will make you happy'.

6. Good Self-Esteem Can Be Obtained By "Self-Affirmation"

This is probably the most familiar 'self-esteem myth' – everyone knows this one, whether they believe it or not. The theory is that if I have low self-esteem it is because I am constantly sending myself negative messages because I am always calling myself stupid, useless, pathetic, etc.

The cure to this unhappy situation – according to the theory – is to send myself positive messages instead, telling myself that I am the opposite of what the negative messages say I am. So I affirm to myself that I am a worthwhile person, that I am as good as everybody else, and so on.

By now it is probably clear what the problem with this simple-minded cure for low self-esteem is. By buying into the self-praise game (self-affirmation game) I am also buying into the self-blame (self-condemnation game). I can't have one without making myself vulnerable to the other.

There is another consideration here too – both self-praise and self-blame are equally meaningless. Anything I say to myself about myself is totally and utterly redundant, which is to say, all 'self-statements' have zero information content.

7. Good Self-Esteem Comes From Being Accepted By Others

If we had said that good self-esteem comes from 'successfully pleasing other people' then it would of course be immediately possible to see the flaw in this. People-pleasing comes out of insecurity.

We also know that it just doesn't work anyway – human nature is such that if you go out of your way to be helpful you are just going to get exploited to the hilt. You won't get any thanks, and what is more, if you ever try to stop being so over-obliging people will get resentful and angry and call you 'selfish'. But to say that good self-esteem comes out of being 'accepted by others' (or perhaps, 'valued by others') doesn't sound so wrong. The only thing is – it is wrong.

Chapter 17
OBSTACLES OF SELF-ESTEEM

I don't know about you but everywhere I look there are barriers to self-esteem. If you are interested in self-development but have low self-esteem, the first thing you need to do is fix that. Until you do, it is much harder to accurately assess what you need to learn and change to achieve your goals. If you have low self-esteem it can be difficult to even see what your goals are.

Imagine yourself as a dartboard. Everything and everyone else around you has the potential to become a damaging dart pin, at one point or another. These dart pins will destroy your self-esteem and pull you down in ways you may not even be conscious of. It's important not to let them destroy you, or get the best of you. So what are the dart pins to avoid, and how can you keep them from hurting you?

Negative Work Environment

Beware of the "Dog eat dog" theory where everyone else is fighting just to get ahead. This is where non-appreciative people usually thrive. No one will appreciate your contributions even if you miss lunch and dinner, and stay up late. You may find you are working harder and harder for less and less in return.

Stay out of this trap, it will ruin your self-esteem. Find ways to manage your work within the normal working day at least 90% of the time. If you have to compete with others, compete on your terms. Do not be drawn into power games or negative behavior that will make you feel bad about yourself.

Other People's Behavior

You will run into bulldozers, brown nosers, gossipmongers, whiners, backstabbers, snipers, the walking wounded, controllers, naggers, complainers, exploders, patronizers and sufferers. All of these negative behaviors in others will damage your self-esteem, as well as to your self-development program. But remember, it is not the person that is the problem: it is their behavior.

Changing Environment

You can't be a green bug on a brown field. Changes challenge our paradigms. They test our flexibility, adaptability, and alter the way we think. Changes will make life difficult for a while and often cause stress, but when we look back we will see that change is often the catalyst or cause of self-development. Try not to resist it.

Past Experience

It's okay to cry and say "ouch!" when we experience pain. But don't let pain transform itself into fear by constantly thinking of the bad things that have happened to you or others in the past. It's easy to wreck a relationship by bringing with you the issues you had in your last relationship and expecting your new partner to be like your previous one. Treat each failure and mistake as a lesson, and move on.

Negative World View

Look at what you're looking at. Don't wrap yourself up with all the negativities of the world. In building self-esteem, we must learn how to make the best out of the worst situations.

Determination Theory

The way you are and your behavioral traits is said to be a mixed end product of your inherited traits, your upbringing, and your current environments such as your friends, your work situation, the economy, and even the climate of the country that you live in.

Do not make the mistake of thinking that your genetics or upbringing will determine how your life goes. You have your own identity. If your father is a failure it doesn't mean you have to be a failure too. Learn from other people's experiences, so you'll never have to encounter the same mistakes.

In life, it's hard to stay firm, especially when things and people around you seem to keep pulling you down. There are many barriers to self-esteem that you can help yourself by protecting yourself from. However, building self-esteem will eventually lead to self-development if we start to become responsible for who we are, what we have, and what we do.

When we develop self-esteem, we take control of our mission, values, and discipline. Self-esteem brings about self-improvement, true assessment, and determination. So how do you start putting up the building blocks of self-esteem? Be positive. Be contented and happy. Be appreciative. Never miss an opportunity to compliment. A positive way of living will help you build self-esteem and set you on the path to positive self-development.

Ways To Overcome The Obstacles Of Self-Esteem:

Self-esteem is a term that describes our overall sense of self-worth or personal value. It is how much we appreciate and like ourselves.

A healthy level of self-esteem can play a significant role in succeeding in life. It means you believe in yourself and are more willing to take chances. But improving self-esteem sometimes requires overcoming various obstacles.

One such obstacle can be waiting for the perfect moment to start or finish something new. To overcome this, it's necessary to live in the present and to take action, rather than waiting for the stars to align perfectly before moving forward. Waiting for things to be "just right" usually means never taking action.

Tied to that can be the belief that we have to be perfect. Instead, it's important to look at our lives as works in progress and to understand that sometimes it's okay to make a mistake or two. It can feel risky to take chances when we can't be positive of the outcome, but when we take that chance, and it comes out well, it means a big boost to our self-esteem and self-confidence.

Another problem in trying to improve self-esteem is that we often ignore our own needs. It can feel good when we do things that please others, but over time it can leave us feeling ignored and not worthy of ourselves. While it's a good thing to be able to offer help to others, our self-esteem increases when our relationships become more reciprocal. When we learn to voice our own needs and to ask for help when it's required, our appreciation of our worth is going to grow as we see that others also value us and are willing to lend a hand.

People with low self-esteem sometimes hide in the background, trying not to be noticed. Doing so can leave us feeling lonely, misunderstood, and frustrated because few people get to know us. The cure is to be willing to share our ideas and opinions and to open ourselves to interactions with more people. Who doesn't feel better about themselves when they have more friends?

Trying something new or even risky is almost always better than staying stuck. But if low self-esteem has you feeling miserable and depressed, and you can't get started on overcoming the problem, consider meeting with a professional counselor who can offer help in working through self-esteem issues.

Follow these steps to overcome the obstacles of self- esteem:

1. Change Your Scenery - Do Something Great And Fun

The way to break a low self-esteem cycle is to do something completely out of the ordinary. It can be as simple as traveling a different route to work in the morning, taking a short weekend vacation to a place you've never visited, or working from a cafe you've always wanted to check out.

Doing something you've never done before or being somewhere you've never been can quickly refresh your mind and break negative thought patterns. We tend to get stuck in a small bubble, neglecting to see that the universe is vast and our problems are usually a lot smaller than we make them out to be.

Changing your scenery can give you a fresh perspective and motivate you to make positive changes rather than dwell in the negative. Give it a shot.

2. Simplify Your Life

Just as our outward appearance is often a reflection of our internal world, our homes are usually a reflection as well. And just as we hold on to negative emotions, beliefs, and thoughts that don't serve us, we often hold on to material possessions that don't serve us either — they weigh us down.

Take a weekend to go through your things and see if you can find some items that might be weighing you down.

Do you have clothes you haven't worn in years? Do you have items that once held sentimental value, but now don't hold the same meaning? What about the things you bought that you thought you'd use, but never have?

Have a yard sale and get rid of those things or donate those items to a local charity. You'll free up some space in your life and in the process, you might just make some money and do something kind for someone else

3. Pursue a Passion

Everyone has a list of things they've wanted to do, but have never got around to doing. We tell ourselves that we don't have the time or money, but we know deep down that we can arrange things in our life to create time or money when it's needed. When you suffer from low self-esteem, you often make excuses as to why you can't pursue your passions, but in the end, it's because you don't believe you deserve to follow your bliss. Stop the cycle and commit to pursuing a passion.

4. Invest in Your Well-Being

Take a look at your spending patterns and see if you can make some changes.

Are you spending money on self-destructive coping mechanisms? Whether it's unhealthy comfort food, excessive drinking, video games or apps, or overindulgence of any kind, these spending habits can be transformed.

By taking the money you spend on indulgences and spending that money on self-improvement, you can empower your mind and body to raise your self-esteem.

Whether it's a retreat, classes, self-improvement courses, hiring a life coach, or simply healthier food, spending money on things that are good for you can make you feel better about yourself.

CONCLUSION

I hope you enjoyed this opportunity to learn about self-esteem! If you take only one important lesson away from this book, make sure it's this one: you absolutely can build your self-esteem, and you can have a big impact on the self-esteem of those you love.

Self-esteem is not a panacea—it will not fix all of your problems or help you sail smoothly through a life free of struggle and suffering—but it will help you find the courage to try new things, build the resilience to bounce back from failure, and make you more susceptible to success.

It is something we have to continually work towards, but it's achievable.

Keep aware of your internal thoughts and external surroundings. Keep focused on your personal goals and all that is possible when self-doubt isn't holding you back.

Stay committed!!!

If you enjoyed this book and you think it will help others, please take a few moments to write a review on your favorite store, and refer it to your friends.

REFERENCES

10 ways to overcome low self-esteem, Deborah Ward, 2 Feb 2020:

https://www.google.com/url?sa=t&source=web&rct=j&url=https://www.psychologies.co.uk/10-ways-overcome-low-self-esteem&ved=2ahUKEwjM6K2Js_ntAhV65-AKHef4DQUQFjAMegQIIRAB&usg=AOvVaw2gUfBASHiz_-kys8xu1jJW

How to Overcome Low Self-Esteem and Negativity, Bonnie Minsky, 22 Oct 2018:

https://www.google.com/url?sa=t&source=web&rct=j&url=https://thriveglobal.com/stories/how-to-overcome-low-self-esteem-and-negativity/&ved=2ahUKEwjM6K2Js_ntAhV65-AKHef4DQUQFjAWegQIIxAB&usg=AOvVaw0y0ixsBH75Eb7VmEd_YTil

6 Self-Love Barriers Holding You Back From Happiness (and How to Overcome Them), Krista Gray, 20 Nov 2018:

https://www.google.com/url?sa=t&source=web&rct=j&url=https://www.brit.co/amp/self-love-barriers-2639487158&ved=2ahUKEwjJ7-bl4PntAhUxDmMBHYeuDtI4ChAWMAJ6BAgJEAE&usg=AOvVaw2MVZ6XPs43dZ3LoqRJNpLE

Practical Tools and Advice to Overcome Low Self Esteem, Self Esteem School.com Website:

https://www.google.com/url?sa=t&source=web&rct=j&url=https://www.self-esteem-school.com/&ved=2ahUKEwjJ7-bl4PntAhUxDmMBHYeuDtI4ChAWMAZ6BAgAEAE&usg=AOvVaw0U4qQIVQuoojXOhU0eG5jV

Self-Esteem, Psychologytoday.com Website:

https://www.google.com/url?sa=t&source=web&rct=j&url=https://www.psychologytoday.com/us/basics/self-esteem&ved=2ahUKEwja0r-G4fntAhUU6OAKHWW0Ds8QFjApegQIIBAB&usg=AOvVaw104mrdAA-qMCW75l-SULsx

How to Build Self-Esteem: 5 Tactics to Change How You See Yourself, Kathleen Smith, 5 Jan 2021:

https://www.google.com/url?sa=t&source=web&rct=j&url=https://www.psycom.net/increasing-self-esteem&ved=2ahUKEwicqv2e4fntAhVYD2MBHffMBBA4FBAWMAB6BAgHEAE&usg=AOvVaw1eFU6L5v_XuHpdSuQZzjaf

8 Common Causes of Low Self-Esteem, Amee LaTour:

https://www.google.com/url?sa=t&source=web&rct=j&url=http://www.goodchoicesgoodlife.org/choices-for-young-people/boosting-self-esteem/&ved=2ahUKEwicqv2e4fntAhVYD2MBHffMBBA4FBAWMAV6BAgEEAE&usg=AOvVaw20BHaxQrWESBEk5ATsaf0K

Counseling Testing Services, www.smsu.edu Website:

https://www.google.com/url?sa=t&source=web&rct=j&url=http://www.smsu.edu/resources/webspaces/campuslife/counselingtestingservices/self%2520esteem.pdf&ved=2ahUKEwiG2r_C4fntAhW88uAKHbs8DuM4HhAWMAF6BAgIEAE&usg=AOvVaw3rNnmFNzAZw6m9BNPkYX5q

Self Esteem – Principles of Addiction, 2013:

https://www.google.com/url?sa=t&source=web&rct=j&url=https://www.sciencedirect.com/topics/social-sciences/self-esteem&ved=2ahUKEwiG2r_C4fntAhW88uAKHbs8DuM4HhAWMAR6BAgAEAE&usg=AOvVaw1gJC7r9b16vqFjLnWbxieR

The use and misuse of self-esteem, Harvard Health Publishing, June, 2007:

https://www.google.com/url?sa=t&source=web&rct=j&url=https://www.health.harvard.edu/newsletter_article/The_use_and_misuse_of_self-esteem&ved=2ahUKEwiG2r_C4fntAhW88uAKHbs8DuM4HhAWMAV6BAgBEAE&usg=AOvVaw3lQVTduJ42MAHSSIeldjqR

What is Self-Esteem and How Can I Improve Mine? The Cali Institute, 3 Feb, 2020:

https://www.google.com/url?sa=t&source=web&rct=j&url=https://calliinstitute.com/what-is-self-esteem/&ved=2ahUKEwiG2r_C4fntAhW88uAKHbs8DuM4HhAWMAd6BAgCEAE&usg=AOvVaw0mvIhmdy3i1VSCaxc0aPPd

5 ways to build lasting self-esteem, Guy Winch, 2016:

https://www.google.com/url?sa=t&source=web&rct=j&url=https://ideas.ted.com/5-ways-to-build-lasting-self-esteem/amp/&ved=2ahUKEwi97s_M4vntAhWD2-AKHb2eBv84KBAWMAd6BAgGEAE&usg=AOvVaw2r3A7dqoEvyJmpdW4cd3nC

How to Overcome Low Self Esteem, Trudi Griffin, 6 Sept 2020:

https://www.google.com/url?sa=t&source=web&rct=j&url=https://www.wikihow.com/Overcome-Low-Self-Esteem%3Famp%3D1&ved=2ahUKEwjzgrXl4vntAhUE2uAKHZ0GDoEQFjAMegQIIBAB&usg=AOvVaw1u4CDW7ozpNPfmqw9Yu2rr&ampcf=1

A Comprehensive Guide to Overcoming Your Low Self-Esteem, 449recovery.org Website:

https://www.google.com/url?sa=t&source=web&rct=j&url=https://www.449recovery.org/low-self-esteem/&ved=2ahUKEwjzgrXl4vntAhUE2uAKHZ0GDoEQFjAZegQIGRAB&usg=AOvVaw2bOxeBzLeWE8YPG4tsKwAR

Overcoming Low Self-Esteem with Mindfulness, Christa Smith, 10 Nov, 2014:

https://www.google.com/url?sa=t&source=web&rct=j&url=https://www.psychologytoday.com/us/blog/shift/201411/overcoming-low-self-esteem-mindfulness%3Famp&ved=2ahUKEwjrvJf84vntAhUPmBQKHX8lCMY4ChAWMAB6BAgGEAE&usg=AOvVaw1sEiVmshizQd--eebOLT_4

25 Things To Remember When You Have LOW Self-Esteem, Barrie Davenport, 16 Nov, 2014:

https://www.google.com/url?sa=t&source=web&rct=j&url=https://liveboldandbloom.com/11/self-confidence/low-self-esteem-signs&ved=2ahUKEwjGtvqO4_ntAhWB2-AKHdDrCsw4KBAWMAJ6BAgHEAE&usg=AOvVaw3al6Cab_jeOwB0xJpPC05-

Why Do People Mistake Narcissism for High Self-Esteem?, Scott Kaufman, 3 Dec, 2018:

https://www.google.com/url?sa=t&source=web&rct=j&url=https://blogs.scientificamerican.com/beautiful-minds/why-do-people-mistake-narcissism-for-high-self-esteem/&ved=2ahUKEwjqrNyk4_ntAhUNohQKHXFECos4FBAWMAF6BAgIEAE&usg=AOvVaw3jROwNufLd14feEJYEWkut

Raising low self-esteem, nhs.uk Website:

https://www.google.com/url?sa=t&source=web&rct=j&url=https:// www.nhs.uk/conditions/stress-anxiety-depression/raising-low-self- esteem/&ved=2ahUKEwjqrNyk4_ntAhUNohQKHXFECos4FBAWMA V6BAgFEAE&usg=AOvVaw1sTEblwoRZKZtbIVT83RcE

www.ingramcontent.com/pod-product-compliance
Lightning Source LLC
Chambersburg PA
CBHW050728030426
42336CB00012B/1458